Younger
Fitter
Stronger

Matt Roberts

The Revolutionary 8-week
Fitness Plan for Men

BLOOMSBURY SPORT

LONDON · OXFORD · NEW YORK · NEW DELHI · SYDNEY

BLOOMSBURY SPORT
Bloomsbury Publishing Plc
50 Bedford Square, London, WC1B 3DP, UK

BLOOMSBURY, BLOOMSBURY SPORT and the Diana logo are trademarks of
Bloomsbury Publishing Plc

First published in Great Britain 2019
Text copyright © Matt Roberts 2019
Original photography © Grant Pritchard 2019
Images on pages 79, 91 © Getty; images on pages 13, 30, 33 © iStock

Bloomsbury Publishing Plc does not have any control over, or responsibility for, any
third-party websites referred to or in this book. All internet addresses given in this
book were correct at the time of going to press. The author and publisher regret
any inconvenience caused if addresses have changed or sites have ceased to exist,
but can accept no responsibility for any such changes

The information contained in this book is provided by way of general guidance in
relation to the specific subject matters addressed herein, but it is not a substitute
for specialist dietary advice. It should not be relied on for medical, health-care,
pharmaceutical or other professional advice on specific dietary or health needs.
This book is sold with the understanding that the author and publisher are not
engaged in rendering medical, health or any other kind of personal or professional
services. The reader should consult a competent medical or health professional
before adopting any of the suggestions in this book or drawing inferences from it.

The author and publisher specifically disclaim, as far as the law allows, any
responsibility from any liability, loss or risk (personal or otherwise) which is
incurred as a consequence, directly or indirectly, of the use and applications of any
of the contents of this book. If you are on medication of any description, please
consult your doctor or health professional before embarking on any fast or diet.

A catalogue record for this book is available from the British Library

Library of Congress Cataloguing-in-Publication data has been applied for

ISBN: PB: 978-1-4729-6449-6; eBook: 978-1-4729-6446-5

2 4 6 8 10 9 7 5 3 1

Printed and bound in China by C&C Offset Printing Co.

Bloomsbury Publishing Plc makes every effort to ensure that the papers used
in the manufacture of our books are natural, recyclable products made from
wood grown in well-managed forests. Our manufacturing processes conform
to the environmental regulations of the country of origin.

To find out more about our authors and books visit www.bloomsbury.com
and sign up for our newsletters.

Contents

Introduction

Welcome to a book that I hope is going to change your life for the better. In the pages that follow I will let you in on everything I've learned from my decades as a trainer

Look in the mirror and what do you see? In your late 30s, 40s and 50s onwards, it's far from unusual to find yourself confronted with the reflection of a rapidly thickening waistline, unsightly man boobs or 'moobs' and a pronounced paunch. Battling the middle-aged spread and a downward slide in fitness are the main concerns of many of my high-profile and high-flying male clients. Yet my promise to them – and to you – is that it doesn't have to be that way.

It's almost one quarter of a century since I opened my first one-to-one training gym in Mayfair. And, in that time, I've noticed a dramatic shift in attitudes towards ageing and how people expect their bodies to look and perform as they get older. Reaching your mid-40s once meant hanging up your trainers for good, now it likely means investing in a few extra pairs so that you can train for a marathon or triathlon. There has been a quite incredible shift in mindset that has catapulted the 50-plus brigade into completely new territory.

At the same age, their parents and grandparents would have considered it an achievement to stay well. Today's 50- and 60-somethings hit their landmark birthdays and ask 'What else can I do to increase my fitness? How many more physical challenges can I achieve?' Among my own clients, who have an average age of 45, I have seen that the physical demands they make of themselves have morphed and developed into what 30-somethings expected a decade ago.

How has this happened? The reasons are several-fold, but there are certainly links between the rapid expansion of the fitness industry – the availability and range of classes, gyms and trainers – and the corresponding rise in body confidence exhibited by these super-agers. Prior to the 1990s, gym memberships were a novel concept. Fast forward almost three decades and it is the same generation who embraced the first gym classes and who paved the way by hiring personal trainers, who are now entering their fifth and sixth decades of life. Perhaps predictably, they are refusing to let their advancing years get the better of them.

And now I am one of them. My goals have always been to remain as fit and healthy at 45 as I was at 35 and at 50 as I was at 40. I want the same for my clients. Yet in my mid-40s, I faced similar health concerns as any man of my age. I realised that the kind of diet and exercise programme that had worked for me until then wasn't having the same effect. It became harder to keep the pounds at bay and to maintain (and improve) the physique I wanted. I knew something needed to change.

That's why I developed an approach that I believe is ground-breaking. It's based on hard science that addresses the hormonal shifts that occur as men get older. Past our 30s, levels of male hormones including human growth hormone (HGH) and testosterone naturally begin to fall. And, since these are essential for regulating muscle and bone growth, fat levels and metabolism, the effects can be devastating. It becomes harder to build muscle, to burn calories and absorb nutrients from food. The result? Muscles wither away and are replaced by

Matt Says:

I believe you can be as fit in your 40s as you were in your 30s

a layer of body fat that accumulates with intensity around your middle and chest to produce the paunch and moobs characteristic of middle age. You become more tired and stressed, your sex drive plummets and you look and feel older.

Sound familiar? Then you have bought the right book. Within these pages is my secret formula for youthful transformation of body and mind. It is a plan based on cutting-edge science that has proven you can boost levels of the key hormones that usually plummet as men get older. By raising levels of HGH and testosterone through a targeted exercise and diet plan, you can not only improve the way you look and feel but help to slow the ageing process.

My 8-week programme is focused on progressively harder strength and high intensity workouts that stimulate the production of HGH and testosterone, boost muscles and strengthen bones that lose mass as we get older. It works in tandem with a diet designed to boost testosterone and HGH and get you eating more of the foods that science has shown can block the production of the female hormone oestrogen. It's rising oestrogen in men's later years that contributes to fat being deposited in the male chest area (yes, your moobs) and around the middle and there are many natural and healthy foods that help to counter it.

Having tried and tested the regimen on myself and countless male clients, I can confirm it works – and with dramatic results. It's not a quick fix. Effort is required, but provided you are prepared to make it and can give this your undivided attention over the next two months then I can promise that you will shed fat, lose 2-3 inches from your middle and banish those moobs. There are other welcome – if less expected – side-effects. Within eight weeks,

you will also discover your sex drive ramps up, your sleep quality gets better and your energy levels soar. You will feel less anxious and find your posture and powers of concentration are dramatically enhanced. You will notice that even the condition and growth of hair and nails gets better.

Believe me it is worth the effort. At 50 you can now expect to live for another 20-30 years. In the half century between 1960 and 2010, the average life span increased by around 10 years for a man and eight years for a woman according to the Office for National Statistics (ONS). Men and women in England are expected to live 79.5 and 83.1 years respectively. Rather than grow old gradually and gracefully, people are grabbing the opportunity to use their spare time and money on maintaining the fitness levels they have fought hard to achieve. And, as science uncovers findings about how we can control the performance and recovery process through balanced training, diet and recovery techniques as we age, it makes super-fitness accessible to us all.

We are entering an era of greater emphasis on maintaining and improving fitness as we get older than ever before. In the Worldwide Survey of Fitness Trends for 2018, published in the *American College of Sports Medicine's Health and Fitness Journal* and based on responses from 4,133 fitness professionals around the globe, one of the biggest predicted trends of the year ahead is a rise in the number of 60-plus-year-olds going to gyms.

And what better motivation is there than the growing number of male celebrities who are able to flaunt the kind of physique that would be envied by the average 30-year-old? From Brad Pitt to George Clooney, they have shown that your 50s are a decade in which you can look as good as you did 20 years previously. We live in an image-obsessed age and there is living proof that even in your 60s and 70s – think Bruce Willis and Sylvester Stallone – you can achieve enviable levels of muscle tone and leanness. Celebrities are famous and fabulous-looking, but physiologically no different to the rest of us. If they can set about preserving youth through exercise and diet, so can you.

My belief is that we can all become super-agers and that you can change a huge amount through the diet, fitness and recovery regimen outlined in these pages. Don't get me wrong, it doesn't come easily and you need to work for it. My super-fit, 40- to 60-plus-something clients don't look great through putting their feet up. They are diligent about their workout routines. There are many factors that come into play as you get older – changes to levels of hormones,

muscle and bone mass that occur naturally with ageing – that make it more challenging to stay in shape. But it is achievable for anyone.

Over the next few chapters, I will take you through the fascinating science that underpins the theories behind my approach. It's worth reading, but if you don't have the time (or the inclination), then head straight to the 'Speed Reads' at the end of each chapter. Once you have familiarised yourself with the basic facts, you can push on with pursuing the results you are after. I am now holding back the years myself and can confirm that it is not only possible to maintain your fitness level and physique as you get older, but to improve it. You too can look and feel as good as you did in your 20s and 30s. Let's get started.

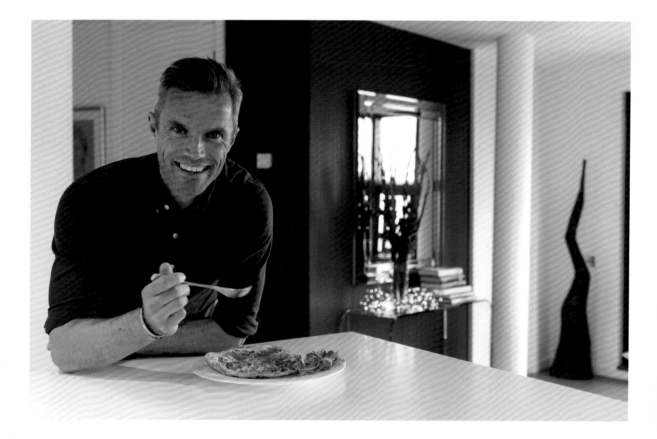

→ Benefits of the 8-week Plan

My promise to you is that you can achieve the following:

1_Weight loss
You will dramatically change your appearance, losing your paunch, moobs, love handles and middle-age spread, achieving the kind of body you had (or wanted) in your 20s

2_Improved sleep
Restless nights will be replaced with hours of restorative sleep

3_Muscle mass
Halt the decline in muscle that occurs after the age of 30 for a stronger, better performing – and better looking – body

4_Hair and nails
Watch as the condition of your hair and nails improve

5_Sex drive
Your libido will soar as you follow the programme

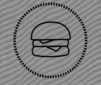

6_Appetite
Hunger pangs and cravings will disappear thanks to a targeted plan that will probably see you eating more calories than before, yet with visible improvements to your physique

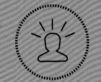

7_Stress
Discover how to halt the rise in stress hormones that can leave you riddled with anxiety

8_Heart health
By boosting your muscle mass, you'll increase your metabolism, improve the efficiency with which your body controls blood sugar, and reduce the likelihood of deadly conditions such as diabetes and stroke.

9_Focus
Watch as your levels of concentration soar, leaving you better able to focus at work

10_Self-confidence
Find yourself reaching new highs as you set – and achieve – goals you once thought impossible

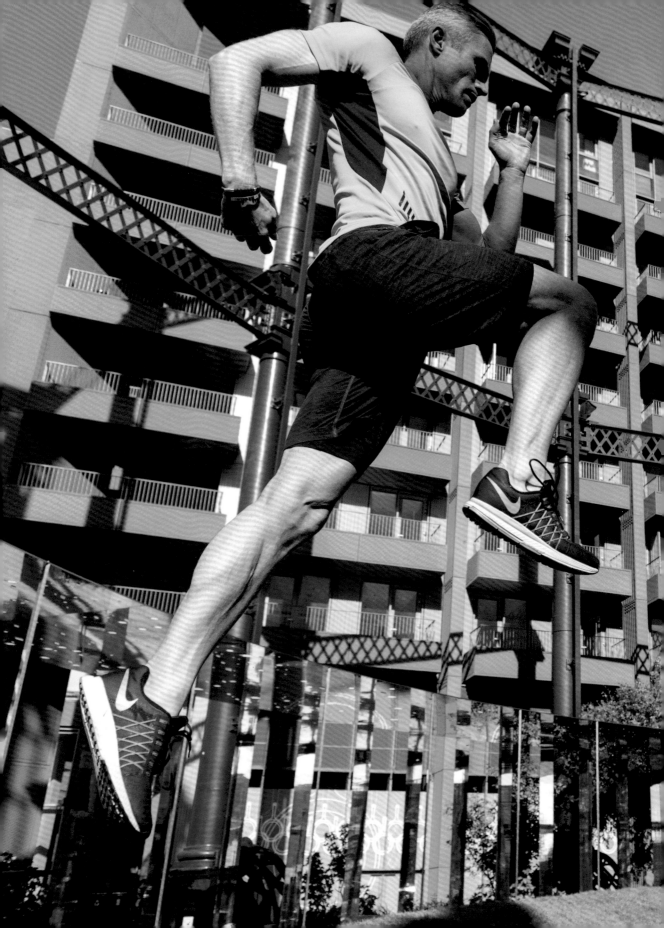

The Science

Before we get down to the practical side of the plan, it is really important that you have an understanding of the basic science underpinning it.

This is not some faddy approach that has short-lived effects. It is based on hard evidence from hundreds of scientific research papers and it is designed to make you look and feel younger, fitter and stronger – not just now, but for the rest of your life.

Men and Women are Different

Our hormones shape who we are and how we function. And male hormones influence everything from your sex drive to your appearance, and from your fitness to your longevity.

Biologically, men and women differ because of the hormones they produce. For years, scientists have known the profound influence hormones have on a woman's health. From childhood through to puberty, childbirth to the menopause, there is documented evidence – and any woman will back it up – that changing levels of the predominantly 'female' sex hormones, including oestrogen, oestradiol, oestriol and oestrone, profoundly affect everything from mood to weight and appearance to health.

Less frequently discussed are the effects of hormones on men, yet we too are influenced by them from our conception. Male hormones are needed to turn a foetus with a Y chromosome into a boy and then have the effect of 'masculinising' the male body and brain. That first rush of the hormone occurs in the womb but is followed by surges during puberty and early adulthood. Remember the cracking and deepening of your voice, the emergence of fluffy facial hair and spots that plagued your early adolescence? All were linked to the flood of male hormones beginning to exert their influence on your developing body. And those hormones, ebbing and flowing as they do throughout our life, have a profound impact on our how we look and feel, our energy levels and our sex drive, our metabolism and our waistlines.

What is testosterone?

In men, it is the so-called male sex hormones that shape their physique, behaviour and health. Specifically, men produce 10-20 times as much of one such chemical, testosterone, as women. It is known as the 'he hormone', associated as it is with increasing a man's sex drive, boosting strength and influencing personality traits related to power and dominance. Derived from cholesterol, testosterone is a steroid hormone – called an androgen – that is responsible for many important bodily functions. It is secreted predominantly by a man's testicles and while women's ovaries and adrenal glands also make it, they do so in much smaller amounts. It's a misconception that, as they develop, men have high levels of testosterone and women have none. Our chemical balance is far more intricate and delicate than that, ebbing and flowing through the decades. A man's body converts some testosterone into oestradiol, a female hormone, and a woman's body has testosterone receptors that are important for many aspects of survival. What differs starkly is the amount of each we produce. In a typical man's body, there will be 3000 to 1000 nanograms of testosterone per decilitre of plasma. In a woman's, just 40 to 60 nanograms.

Yet even on a daily basis, hormone levels fluctuate, with researchers suggesting that testosterone rises through the night, peaking first thing at around 8 a.m. and then declining again throughout the day reaching its lowest around 8 p.m. The peaks and troughs are more considerable for the under-40s compared to those in their 60s and 70s. And all sorts of things can change the shift in either direction. As you will find out in the coming pages, your diet, lifestyle, stress levels and exercise habits all influence your hormone levels on a daily basis.

What is Human Growth Hormone?

Testosterone and other male-specific hormones don't act alone. There are other chemicals responsible for much of what happens to our bodies as we mature into adults. Among them is Human Growth Hormone (HGH), or somatotropin,

Matt Says:

Hormone levels are influenced by your diet, stress levels, exercise habits and lifestyle

a protein naturally produced by the pituitary gland, responsible for stimulating growth of tissues throughout the body. During adolescence HGH triggers the growth of bone and cartilage. And throughout life it works to boost protein production, enhances the body's utilisation of fat, and influences blood sugar levels. Its production is controlled by a complex set of hormones in the hypothalamus area of the brain and in the intestinal tract and pancreas and, rather cleverly, HGH is released in bursts as a response to different stimuli. When you exercise, experience trauma or sleep, HGH levels are hiked.

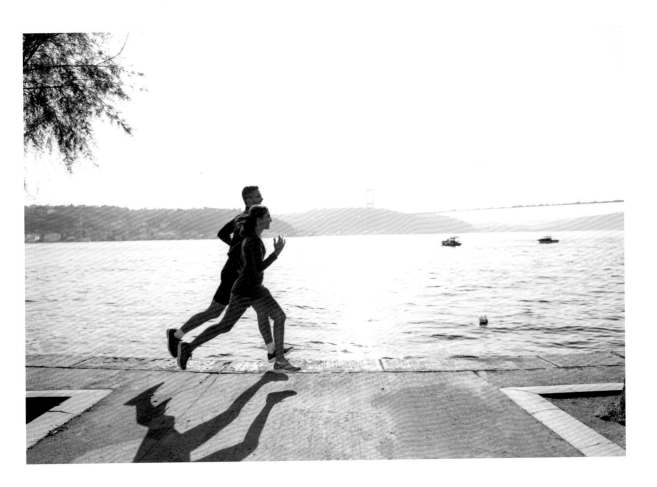

The Hormonal Decline

As we get older, our hormone levels begin to drop, a change that has the potential to affect our health, wellbeing and fitness, but also the way we look

The hormonal tidal wave that occurs in our first three decades of life doesn't last forever. From around the age 30, production starts to wane. Men lose testosterone at an alarming rate of 1.5 to 2 per cent per year once they hit the age of 30 and, simultaneously, the body's growth-hormone production declines and continues to fall. Sometimes there are clear medical reasons for a sharper than average decline. Low testosterone can occur when one or both testicles are damaged, as a side effect of certain medications, or due to a genetic defect. It can also be the result of cancer in the pituitary gland, a tiny organ near the base of the brain that releases a compound called luteinising hormone. Luteinising hormone gives the testicles their testosterone-producing orders and without it the sex-hormone production slows or stalls.

But there is evidence, too, that men today generally have lower testosterone levels than a generation ago. And that our lifestyles are partly to blame. One US study [1] published around a decade ago suggested there had been a 'substantial' drop in men's testosterone levels since the 1980s, with a 60-year-old man in 2004 having testosterone levels 17 per cent lower than those of a man of the same age in 1987. Another paper [2], by Danish scientists, showed that men born in the 1960s – the current crop of 50-somethings – had experienced double-digit declines in hormone levels compared to those born in the 1920s. And in statistics produced by the College of Endocrinology, it was suggested that today's 30-year-old males have 20 per cent less testosterone in their bodies than men 20 years ago. What's causing this mass decline is not fully understood, but experts suspect our diets – more sugar and alcohol, fewer fresh foods and vegetables – and other factors such as long working hours, stress and lower levels of physical activity are playing a part.

Real risks

In addition to the downturn in appearance, sex drive and your body's health and function, there are very real health risks to plummeting hormone levels. At the University of Michigan [3], it was shown how dwindling total testosterone levels in men may be associated with chronic disease, even among men 40 years of age and younger. Using data from the National Health and Nutrition Examination Survey, the Michigan team examined the extent to which low testosterone (low-T) – called hypogonadism – is prevalent among men of all ages. They found that low total testosterone was associated with death from two or more chronic conditions in all age groups, but that it was more prevalent among men with testosterone deficiency.

Men with low testosterone are also more likely to suffer low mood or depression. This was demonstrated in a paper produced by the Center for Andrology at the George Washington University School of Medicine and Health Sciences [4]. Of 200 adult men, with an average age of 48, who were referred with low testosterone levels, 56 per cent had

Matt Says:

With low testosterone, you are more likely to suffer low mood

→ The Declining Body

Dwindling levels of male hormones can take a devastating toll on our bodies. Here are some of the side-effects of hormone levels plummeting:

1_Muscle loss

From our mid-30s we lose muscle mass through a process known as sarcopenia. Do nothing to slow the rate of decline and an average 90g of muscle is lost each year from the age of 40, with men experiencing a sharper decline than women. By the age of 50 you could be losing up to 500g of muscle a year. By the time you are in your 70s you will typically have a third less muscle mass than you did at your strongest. Common complaints include 'not feeling as strong' as you did and failing to become more muscular despite going to the gym.

2_Moobs

Drops in testosterone and rising oestrogen contribute to fat being deposited in the male chest area – and the development of unsightly male boobs or 'moobs'.

3_Love handles

Shifting hormones also means that fat tends to settle as love handles around your midriff. Your body becomes more sensitive to sugars as you reach your 40s, 50s and 60s, or as your fitness levels fall — factors that often coincide – which exacerbates the accumulation of middle fat.

3_Paunch

A complex interplay of hormones in middle age causes the notorious male paunch, a risk factor for heart disease and strokes. Researchers have long suspected that a protruding belly is linked to lower testosterone among men, but the latest evidence suggests that the so-called female hormone oestrogen also plays a role [5]. Why? Testosterone is converted into oestrogen when it breaks down in the body, so decreasing levels of testosterone in men also lead to a higher total proportion of oestrogen. And researchers who compared men with exactly the same levels of testosterone, but different levels of oestrogen, found it was their high levels of oestrogen that were linked to the accumulation of body fat around the middle.

4_Hair loss

Hair loss has long been linked to virility, a consequence of the belief that men with high levels of testosterone are more likely to lose their hair, especially if baldness runs in the family. In fact, baldness in men is caused when hair follicles become exposed to too much dihydrotestosterone (DHT), a chemical synthesised from the male hormone testosterone that binds to receptors in your scalp. By boosting your testosterone levels, as you will with my plan, you will help to prevent hair loss.

Less facial hair

Facial hair is regulated by testosterone production. Low levels cause males to lose this hair, so very often the first sign of plummeting testosterone is when you find you need to shave less frequently.

Do find you are shaving less than you used to?

6_Sleep problems

Normal testosterone production requires restful, undisturbed sleep. Older men who gradually get fewer hours of sleep each night will therefore experience a gradual lowering of testosterone. As testosterone levels go down, the stress hormone cortisol increases, resulting in shallower and shorter sleep. The hormone-sleep link is complex (see chapter 7), but essentially it's a vicious circle: the less testosterone you have, the more trouble you will have sleeping, and the worse your sleep patterns are, the less testosterone you will produce. In a 2011 study [6], ten young men volunteered to have their testosterone levels measured over a period of eight days in which they were only allowed five hours of sleep per night, far less than they were used to getting. Results showed that day-time testosterone levels dropped by 10 to 15 per cent as a result of their sleep deprivation. The lowest testosterone levels were in the afternoon and evening. Understandably, their energy levels also dropped.

7_Night sweats

It's not just women who experience night sweats as a result of hormonal flux from middle age onwards. Changing hormone levels are a common cause of night sweats in men. A lack of testosterone means false signals are sent to the hypothalamus in the brain, prompting a night sweat. High levels of stress and a lack of fitness can exacerbate the problem.

9_Reduced semen volume

Since testosterone is required to produce a normal ejaculatory volume of 1.5-5 millilitres, men with low levels often report that semen volume seems lower than normal.

10_Shrinkage

Both your penis and testicles can shrink because surplus testosterone is not available to maintain their size and function. Testicles often feel softer and smaller in size.

11_Genital numbness

According to researchers, many men with lowering levels of male hormones can experience slight numbness in the genital area and a failure to respond to touch.

12_Brain decline

As hormone levels decline, so too might your ability to concentrate and focus. Studies show that older men with depression tend to have testosterone levels that are nearly 20 per cent lower than normal [8] and researchers have also shown that low levels of the hormone increased the risk of Alzheimer's disease in men, even when other risk factors for dementia were considered [9]. Conversely, higher levels of testosterone in middle-aged men have been linked to the preservation of brain tissue in many regions of the brain later in life. However, naturally boosting levels is key. Oxford researchers reported [10] that both low levels of testosterone and excessively high levels of testosterone may result in a decrease in cognitive function, so exercise and diet are the best boosters.

Snoring

Obstructive sleep apnoea is a condition in which breathing becomes obstructed during sleep. Symptoms, including loud snoring and breathing problems, are common in men as they age and have been linked to lower levels of male hormones. A 2012 study [7] found men with sleep apnoea were almost 50 per cent more likely to have low testosterone than men without the condition.

depression or depressive symptoms. One quarter of the men in the study were taking antidepressants and had high rates of obesity and low rates of physical activity. Other symptoms included erectile dysfunction, decreased libido, fewer morning erections, low energy and insomnia.

What can be done?

'Are you sad and/or grumpy?' and 'Are you falling asleep after dinner?' These are typical questions being asked by pharmaceutical companies selling testosterone products, which have become the therapy of choice for some men looking to defy the downhill slide of maleness, previously considered an unavoidable side-effect of getting older. Men, it seems, can't get enough of the 'he' hormone in synthetic form and, as demand rises, so a multibillion-pound industry is being spawned.

Although NHS prescriptions are available for extreme cases of low-T, it is private prescriptions fuelling the boom. Global sales of testosterone replacement products now exceed £1.35 billion

and the pharmaceutical industry is putting huge amounts into developing injectables, gels and patches. In America, the advertising tracker Kantar Media estimates that spending on ads for testosterone products has nearly tripled in the last few years.

But while drugs and chemical intervention are sometimes necessary for medical reasons, they are not the answer for the vast majority of men. There are natural ways that you can re-boot HGH and male hormones to look and feel your best, namely in the form of diet and exercise, sleep and recovery.

Although some supplements (see chapter 3) can aid hormone maintenance, my belief is that much can be done by eating the right foods. Coupled with a lifestyle that nurtures your hormonal status rather than destroys it, I am certain that you can help to slow the effects of ageing without resorting to medication.

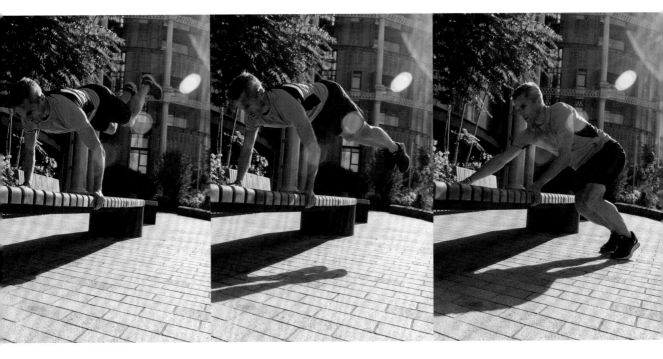

The Power of Exercise

There is little doubt that exercise is key to anti-ageing. We now know that regular exercise affects the body at a cellular level, protecting it against the ravages of time in a host of different ways

One example of how activity helps is the way exercise affects the cells' telomeres, the tiny caps found on the end of DNA strands that are thought to protect against damage. As we age, those telomeres shorten and fray. It's a natural process, but one that is accelerated by obesity, smoking, inactivity, stress and a lack of sleep, all of which cause cells to age.

Several studies have shown that athletes in their 60s and 70s have much longer telomeres than sedentary people of the same age, but a notable study [11] conducted a few years ago suggested the same effect is true when anyone of any age exercises. Using information gleaned from the US National Health and Nutrition Examination Survey, involving tens of thousands of adults who provided information about their lifestyles and a blood sample, researchers from the University of Mississippi and University of California set about comparing exercise habits of the participants with the telomere length of their white blood cells. The anti-ageing association was clear from the results.

In the study each person was given a single point for taking part in an activity – weight training, moderate exercise such as walking, more vigorous exercise such as running, or walking or cycling to work – during a stated month. Someone who took part in a single activity, so earning one point, was about 3 per cent less likely to have very short telomeres than someone who did nothing. And the improvements were more dramatic among those who were most active. If people had taken part in two types of exercise, they were 24 per cent less likely to have short telomeres; those who did three types of exercise were 29 per cent less likely. Those who ran, cycled, swam and walked, for example, and those who had participated in all four types of activities were 59 percent less likely to have very short telomeres.

And the best news for those of you who have bought this book? The strongest links between exercise and telomere improvement occurred between the ages of 40 and 65, suggesting it's never too late to act.

Hormonal boost

The right combination of activity also stems hormonal decline and can boost levels of the hormones men need most to preserve body and mind. When we are physically active, our motor neurons, or nerve cells that supply your muscle fibres, increase thereby triggering neurotransmitters to release hormones. Levels of HGH released from the anterior pituitary gland also spike during exercise. And, in the long term, the age-defying benefits can be vast. However, boosting levels of HGH and testosterone is not as straightforward as going at it hard and long in the gym. It is important to train not just in the right way, but for an appropriate duration. Workouts need to be controlled and progressive to achieve the desired results and, crucially, must be combined with a tailored dietary approach.

Matt Says:

Levels of growth hormones spike when we do the right sort of exercise

Types of Exercise

There is no single type of exercise that will restore your hormonal balance. However, some types should have a greater emphasis than others in your workouts

The type and quantity of exercise you do is hugely important and I have created a programme that maximises results. Here are the types of exercise you will be doing (along with those you won't):

Resistance training

Working against a resistance – including weight training - is essential to offset the downturn in hormones and muscle mass that occur with age. Partly this is down to the effects of resistance training on HGH and testosterone. As long as three decades ago, exercise scientists at Ball State University's Human Performance Laboratory found that 'strength training can induce growth hormone and testosterone release, regardless of age' [12]. Since then, it's something that has been studied extensively by world leading experts, among them Stuart Phillips, Professor of Kinesiology at McMaster University, Canada. For one study [13], funded by the Natural Sciences and Engineering Research Council of Canada, Phillips and his team recruited 49 young men who had been weight training for a year or more and put them through a battery of tests of their strength, fitness, hormone levels and muscular health. All of the volunteers then performed three sets of weight training lifts four times per week for 12 weeks, some with heavier weights, others lighter. By the end of the three-month trial, all of the men had gained muscle strength and size, and all had more testosterone and HGH flowing through their bodies after the training sessions.

There are reams of other evidence to support this spike in hormones both immediately after a strength session and longer term. If weight training has been overlooked in your own exercise routine, now is the time to add it. I'll be taking you through some resistance training exercises step by step later on in the book.

Metabolic circuits

In the programme you will be following, I have included metabolic or 'Met' training, a high intensity approach to circuit training that primes your body for enhanced hormonal response. This type of training is fast, intense and hard work, but has been shown in studies [14] to stimulate the production of HGH, which slows down aging by increasing exercise capacity, increasing bone density, increasing muscle mass, and decreasing body fat. This type of intense training in overweight adults boosts levels of brain-derived neurotrophic factor (BDNF), which has been dubbed 'Miracle-Gro® for the brain' and linked to improved executive functioning and memory.

Endurance exercise

Some light cardio exercise can enhance hormone production. It's certainly something I advocate in my training programmes. For two studies [15, 16], scientists at King's College London and the University of Birmingham recruited 125 amateur cyclists aged 55 to 79, 84 of whom were male and 41 of whom were female. The participants underwent a series of laboratory tests and were compared to a group of adults who did no regular physical activity. Results showed cyclists in the study didn't gain excess body fat as they got older and their cholesterol levels were not raised. In the male cyclists, levels of testosterone — which would usually have dwindled with the passing years — remained high.

Beware the tipping point

Train for endurance events within your body's capacity and testosterone falls and then, during the recovery period over the next few days, it recovers to higher levels. But overdoing long bouts of traditional cardio can actually damage your mitochondria and accelerate aging. And for men in middle age who repeatedly push their bodies to the extremes of multi-marathons, ultra-endurance runs or triathlons on a regular basis, low testosterone can occur as a consequence of overtraining [17].

Placing your body under more stress than it can handle sends levels of the so-called stress hormone, cortisol, into overdrive and, in turn, can hinder your body's testosterone production. Endless miles on foot or on the bike is also more likely to lead to very low body-fat percentages that can also play a role in testosterone loss. Fat cells produce the hormone called leptin, responsible for telling the brain that you have enough food to avoid starvation, and when those messages aren't received, the brain cuts off the production of sex hormones in a bid to conserve energy for survival.

Extreme levels of endurance training can play havoc with your hormones. Indeed, the elite American marathon runner, Ryan Hall, says he was forced to end his career abruptly as a result of his own testosterone levels plummeting. For 20 years, Hall had kept his weekly mileage steadily above 100 miles, a regime that led to him recording a time of 2 hours 4 minutes 58 seconds in the 2011 Boston Marathon. Yet, in 2016, he revealed that his chronically low testosterone levels had caused a fatigue so extreme he was barely able to cover 12 gentle running miles a week [18].

Matt Says:

True fitness is the balance of strength, mobility, endurance, stamina and stability

It seems that, in the case of Hall and others, oxidative damage and inflammation of muscles leads to the release of cytokines, proteins that produce fatigue, low mood and other side-effects, which eventually take their toll. There's some evidence that these cytokines also increase tryptophan levels in the brain, altering the serotonin metabolism, which is closely related to fatigue. With the right combo of exercise, rest and refuelling – as outlined in my programme – this will be avoided. Your body will thrive, recover and rebuild with phenomenal effect.

Speed Read

→ Chemicals including testosterone, a male hormone, and Human Growth Hormone (HGH) are essential for strength, masculinity and a youthful appearance.

→ Levels of testosterone and HGH start to decline in men from our mid-30s onwards.

→ Side-effects of hormonal decline include weight gain, an unsightly paunch and moobs, along with poor sleep patterns and memory loss.

→ Exercise and diet help to stem hormonal losses.

→ Resistance training and metabolic circuits are key – along with some aerobic activity.

→ Your brain – and memory – can be enhanced through a carefully planned workout regimen.

→ Too high a volume of exercise – and overtraining – can accelerate ageing.

→ Brain Gains

Fit body, fit mind has never been more true. We are continually seeing new, well-researched evidence of how exercise and physical well-being play a vital role in mental health

It's not just your muscles that will benefit from the resistance training you will be including in your exercise regimen. Science has proven that strength gains correlate with improved neurological health – in other words your brain power is enhanced along with your physique and lifespan. Of course, the concept of physical strength being linked to mental power is nothing new. It's something the ancient Greeks firmly believed and a reason why ancient Greek philosophers, including Aristotle, used weight training as a means to aid thinking. And researchers have since proven they really were onto something.

A recent UK study involving 324 healthy female identical twins, aged between 43 and 73, put one twin on a leg-strength training programme but not the other. At the end of the 10-year trial, results published in the journal *Gerontology* [19] showed a striking 'protective relationship' between muscle power and cognitive improvement.

Another paper [20], in 2016, by a team of Australian researchers also looked at the effects of weight training on brain health. Working with 68 women and 32 men aged 55 to 86, all of whom had mild cognitive impairment, the scientists from the Centre for Healthy Brain Ageing (CHeBA) at the University of New South Wales and the University of Adelaide asked one group to perform weight training twice a week for six months, lifting 80 per cent of their maximum capacity, and the other group to do stretching exercises. In this Study of Mental and Resistance Training (SMART) trial, cognitive tests performed at the start and end of the trial and 12 months after the study revealed that the weight training group scored significantly higher at the end of the study than at the beginning and retained those improvements a year later. However, the scores of the stretching group had declined somewhat. It backed up previous findings from the same team who had used MRI scans to show an increase in the size of specific areas of the brain among those who took part in a weight training program.

Why this happens had been a source of mystery, even to the world's most eminent scientists. However, they are much closer to understanding how and why strength training affects the brain in a positive way. In 2018, Italian scientists reported [21] that neurogenesis (the growth of new nerve cells and connections in the body) is impaired when animals don't do load-bearing exercise, the kind that involves moving against a resistance. When resistance training is performed, the mitochondria, or power house of a cell, in the large muscles of the legs are wired to send beneficial proteins to the brain. When load-bearing exercise is ignored, these proteins aren't generated in sufficient quantities. The result? Neurological growth and brain function suffer.

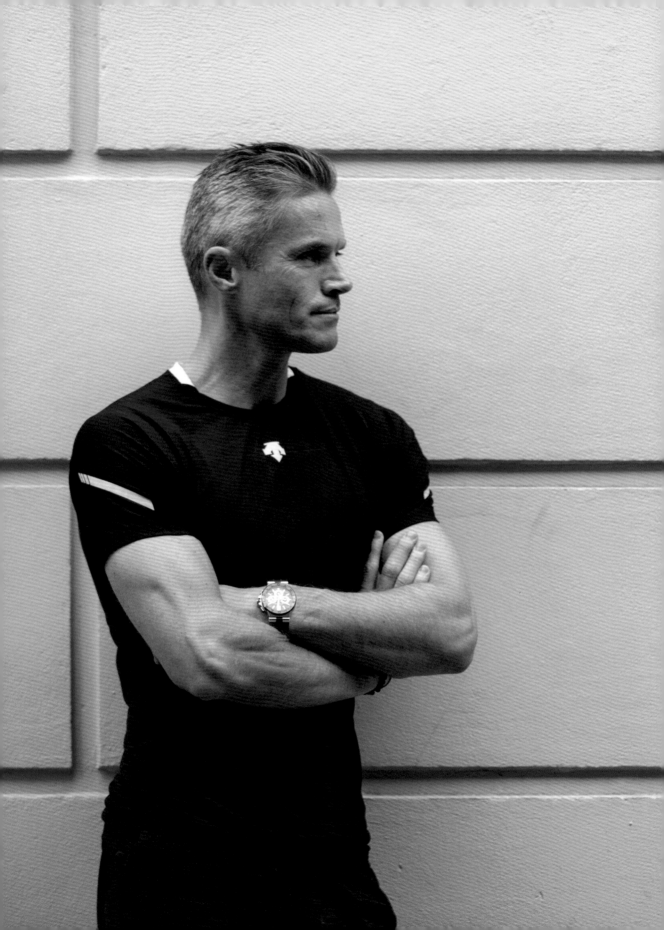

Chapter Two

How the Plan Works

Now we are getting stuck in to the detail of what lies ahead. In this section I will be outlining the areas of your life that will need addressing in order to slow the ageing process. You will learn not just about why you need to change the way you eat and exercise, but also about the importance of sleep, recovery and digestive health. I promise it is not as daunting as it might sound. Read on …

8 Weeks to a Better You

All of the methods I employ with my clients – and with you – have been tried and tested many times and are the subject of scientific study. They can change your life for the better.

My 8-week programme is revolutionary. It is designed to be kind to the ageing male body while restoring it to its prime. But the goal, the aim and the success of this programme is measured by one key thing: *you* should feel like the very best version of *you* when you have completed it.

This principle underpins the way I train anyone – from A-listers to high-fliers. I am always looking for the best ways in which to ensure that my clients are happy, fulfilled and self-confident. As we get older, our view of ourselves, of our environment, our relationships and careers, can change. Whether this is down to these things fundamentally changing in themselves or whether it is our perception of them changing is somewhat subjective, but it is fair to assume that, if we have a lower level of self-respect, our view of the world around us will be a little more jaded.

What's certain is that when we don't feel like the best version of ourselves, we behave differently. When we are tired, we can become snappier or perhaps less decisive. When we feel physically out of shape or overweight, we are perhaps less inclined to be outgoing and open. When stiffness, aches and pains are a conscious presence as we wake up, when we exercise or just when we move around during the day, our sense of vulnerability is heightened and our limitations magnified. If these things are happening because we've let our well-being habits slip for a while, we might feel that they can be rectified. But if they are a direct result of us either a) thinking we are ageing or b) actually ageing and doing nothing to fully help ourselves, then our sense of self-purpose, optimism and vitality will take a hammering.

What I'm promising is that you will find a way to optimise your body, and you will find a way to stop the body from slowing down, aching, changing shape and losing energy, not just in your mid-30s but in your 40s, 50s, 60s and beyond. I believe we can all feel like the very best versions of ourselves and achieve greater and greater things on a daily basis for many years to come.

This programme is designed to be used in a specific way, based on a large number of different scientific studies, research data and practical experience. My company has delivered more than a million hours of personal training over the years it has been trading, which has been a perfect test bed for the work that we do, allowing us to refine, tweak and perfect the solution. This is the result.

It will require an open mind if you are used to pounding out endless miles on your bike or in your trainers, but the results will speak for themselves. I've observed my clients transform their bodies on this programme and now I am hoping to help you do the same. Within weeks you will notice that body fat levels diminish and you begin to look more toned. After two months on the programme you could find your waist narrows by 2-3 inches and your moobs miraculously disappear, you are energised and your libido soars. What more could you want?

So how does it work? Within the overall programme, there are different areas of 'training' that you need to embrace in order to maximise results. These five 'gateways' or 'factors to success', as I like to call them, are essential if you really want to achieve the goals I've been outlining. To achieve success as quickly as possible all five gateways or factors need to be improved. Here's how:

Factor One

Exercise

How much and of what type of physical activity you do on a daily and weekly basis has a huge bearing on your hormone levels and your overall wellbeing

Of course, this is a major player in my 8-week programme and, by the end of it, I promise you will achieve the following key goals:

→ You will look and feel 'cosmetically' fit.
→ You will have stronger muscles and strong functional movement patterns.
→ Your bone structure and strength will improve.
→ You will have better cardiovascular conditioning, speed and agility.
→ Your body will be more mobile and less prone to joint pain and strain or injuries.

The plan has some surprises. Out are the lengthy cardio sessions and repeated hardcore HIIT that really take their toll when you are in your 40s and 50s, leaving you prone to overuse injuries; in come strength sessions designed to produce the growth hormones that will leave you looking and feeling younger. The emphasis will be on developing pure strength in all the major compound movements. My aim is to help you to maximise the hypertrophy effect within your upper body to give it shape and definition. But you'll also work bi-laterally and uni-laterally to improve balance and all-over mobility.

Matt Says:

Don't let your age change the way you think about yourself. Keep pushing yourself to achieve new goals

As we have seen in chapter 1, there's no shortage of scientific evidence that this is the ideal approach for men of our age. Weight training builds muscle and power; it strengthens your skeleton and improves your physique. And it does this largely through priming your hormonal system to release increased levels of testosterone and growth hormone following a strength-based workout session.

There is a caveat – this level of training must be balanced with good nutrition and with rest and recovery. A lot of middle-aged men find they sleep less well than they used to and it's a direct result of their adrenal glands being constantly drained by the strain of work and unnecessarily long gym sessions, so don't neglect the four remaining 'gateways' of my programme.

Everyday stretches

On days when you are not working out, I suggest you do some of the everyday stretches I've outlined on pages 98–99. These will really help to keep you mobile and to ensure you are ready to work hard again the following day.

Activation drills

Prior to every session you will be asked to perform some activation exercises. 'What are these?' you may be wondering. Well, very few of the movements we perform involve a solitary muscle. Whenever we move we are trying to coordinate a number of muscles to work in a given sequence to make sure that we complete the entire movement, don't over-strain the body in making that movement, and don't overload any one muscle group to complete that move.

Our aim is to train the body to have a better balance of muscle use. Let's use an example of the glutes or buttock muscles. I often see clients who come to me in a state where their glutes are under-used as they don't use these muscles enough when walking, standing, sitting, getting up, getting down and even when exercising. This chronic under-use of the muscles tends to result in over-use of, and therefore strain on, the muscles of the lower back and the hips and front of thighs. If allowed to continue, this will lead to pain and injury.

That's where activation drills come in. I use them within my programme to fire up many of these secondary muscles that are so important in large movements. By activating these muscles before you get to the main 'bigger' exercises you are effectively preparing them for the work ahead.

Pre-workout mobility drills

In addition to activation exercises, your preparation for each workout will include mobility drills or pre-workout mobilisers. Why do I advocate using these? Mobility is important for all of us. The ability to move well and be able to perform all movement patterns cannot be underestimated, especially as we get older.

When I talk about mobility what I am actually talking about is the relationship between the muscles and the bones and the stress put on the bones by tight or weak muscles. This stress has an effect on our ability to move joints through the required range, which has an effect on the way we physically move. We are all born with a great range of mobility; nurture not nature makes us lose it. If you spend much of the day sitting at a desk, the likelihood is that you will have shortened hip flexors and hamstrings, which places stress through the lower back and hips and also limits movement. For this reason, I encourage everyone to make mobility work part of their daily routine. Stretching, mobility drills and soft tissue drills all help to make sure that we move well, reduce the risk of joint pain and feel younger. The aim is to free up tight muscles and create better movement in every joint. By doing this before we move onto our more loaded exercises, it also helps to ensure a better, less restricted movement, which in turn reduces the risk of injury from the loaded exercises.

When doing the mobility drills and soft tissue work aim to really feel the work you are doing rather than just going through the motions. In areas of tightness, work that little longer to try and release the restriction. All the mobility drills can be done at any time and always help to keep us moving better.

Lifting

With every repetition and every weight lifted, I want you to focus on the quality of each movement. What we will be aiming to do is to overload your muscles appropriately so that they respond in a positive way by growing and becoming more defined.

Think power: Focus on the 'power' aspect of the lift. When you lift a weight, there are 'positive' and 'negative' parts of the movement: the positive part is the movement that moves the weight when you push, pull or lift it, and the negative is the phase that returns the weight back to its start position. With a Bench Press, the negative phase is the lowering of the bar towards the chest and the positive is the actual push phase of the movement.

Think pace: I also want you to think about the speed of each lift. Your positive (lifting or pushing) movements should generally take half the time of the negative movements in this programme - a slow 'recoil' and a powerful 'lift'. This explosion of power will allow a significant and controlled overload, maintaining great technique and form, and will produce the optimum payback. Besides the muscle, bone and hormone benefits of this, you will also be at less risk of injury as we are really focusing on using speed that requires great technique at all times.

Think quality: Between groups of sets I want you to be aware of how you are feeling, not just picking a time to do your next set. We achieve overload by doing back-to-back sets with little recovery, followed by a period of almost full recovery. We want quality in every aspect of your training programme. It's not a race. Enjoy the process, enjoy the workouts and be conscious about how your body feels. Training should

→ Daily Structure

Within the programme, you will find five different types of day structure. Below I explain how these days work, and some key terminology

Strength focused: These days focus on mobility and strength, beginning with drills to fine-tune your range of motion and ease structural stiffness. Then you'll focus on strength moves, in isolation or as part of super-sets. You'll finish off with a stretch of the major muscles worked.

Strength plus metabolic finisher: This type of day has the same intent and focus as the strength days, but we add a high intensity finisher. This will raise the metabolism and burn extra calories, long after the workout is over. You have a choice of three finishers; I would suggest that you rotate the finishers each day and, as you get fitter, you can achieve more each time you perform one.

Strength circuits: The aim of these days is to work at medium intensity over a longer duration to achieve strength, endurance and a caloric burn. The exercises in this workout are performed one after another in two different groups. Perform all of group 1 for the stated sets, before moving on to group 2. Move quickly from one exercise to the next. The exercises in this workout will not feel as difficult as those on other days, but the combined effect will make the workout as a whole feel tough.

Rest day: There is no exercise requirement on these days, although that is not to say you should sit around and do nothing! Rest, recover and eat really well to power the active days ahead.

Fasting day: On fasting days, your focus is keeping your diet as clean as possible and making sure that you maintain the eight-hour eating window.

Reps: Every exercise comes with a required rep range. As the programme develops there are different rep requirements depending on whether the focus is strength, muscle building or muscular endurance. In Phase One, you'll find rep ranges of 10-12. The aim here is that you have to push hard over the last 2-3 reps. Once you get further into the programme, the rep ranges become much smaller. At the 3-6 rep ranges, the exercises take more concentration and more work.

Sets: This means the number of times that you will perform the stated number of reps of a given exercise. So if you see '5 reps x 5 sets', this simply means that you perform the exercise for five reps, then rest or move to the next exercise, later returning to this exercise. In this example you will perform the five reps five times.

Supersets: A superset is a combination of two or three exercises that work opposing muscle groups. When you see 'superset', perform the exercises in that superset one after another for the stated number of sets, then move to the next superset.

Tempo: This is the speed at which you move in any stage of a given exercise. We show this as a series of four numbers, for example 2:0:2:0. The first number is the first part of the movement, the second number is the rest period, the third number is the second part of the movement and the fourth number is the rest. In this example the movement is continuous with no rest at any stage. Later in the programme we start to use more 'time under tension', reflected by higher numbers in the tempo.

be 'considered' and not just a frantic blast all the time. Sure, some parts require speed, short recovery and rapid movements, but I want you to be thinking about how each part of this connects together, and about making every part of your body feel good.

Think mobility: You will also be completing regular mobility drills to help improve movement and, if you spend much of your working life deskbound, to prevent making matters worse. These are a really important part of the programme and I urge you not to skip them in the belief that only hardcore weight training matters. Success is a balance of many different factors, and this is one of them.

Think data: The programme also works on metabolic stamina-improving cardiovascular activity to help boost effective fat burning and condition the heart. This needs to be done in a sensible and controlled style that monitors and shows improvements in quality of work and heart rate recovery. Data-rich training that can be charted – a training diary is the simplest method, but you can use trackers and heart rate monitors – is the only way of really showing improvement and pushing motivation.

Limited-rest supersets

Within the programme the focus is first of all on strength improvement, and I have prioritised that as the first part of the workouts. Intensity is important as we get older. Long duration workouts tend to be too fatiguing and therefore the quality reduces. With superset exercises you are able to keep up the intensity by working muscles on one side of the body followed immediately by muscles on the other side. I have also limited total rest time by allowing only a short rest period after both superset exercises have been performed on each set. Working in this way has been proven to have a greater effect on the level of work within the two working muscles groups and therefore create greater micro-damage – or tiny tears - that will lead to greater muscle adaptation and ultimate improvements in strength.

Compound moves

Compound exercises involve large muscle groups and include exercises such as squats, lunges or lateral lunges. They are the very foundation of how we move and require many muscles to co-ordinate to create one big movement. They are immensely important in any exercise programme, but hold particular value for anyone who has purchased this book. Here's why:

They burn more calories. Exercises that involve more muscle tissue require more oxygen, which helps the body increase its net energy expenditure.

They improve muscle coordination. Moving the hips in all three planes of motion enhances the way the muscles work together to produce movement.

They elevate the heart rate. The purpose of cardiovascular exercise is to improve the ability of the heart to function as a pump. You can achieve this through exercise such as running and cycling, or by doing exercises that involve a significant amount of muscle use. Performing a single muscle exercise, such as biceps curls with dumbbells, uses only a limited amount of muscle tissue; these exercises are more appropriate for focusing on isolated strength. Squats to shoulder presses, press-ups and Russian twists are all examples of compound exercises that involve large amounts of muscle use, which force the heart to pump blood to keep the muscles fueled.

They improve cognitive skill. The higher skill level required to create these movements trains the learning part of the brain to understand and store that movement.

They boost mobility. When most people think of mobility they picture static stretching. Yet, any exercise that involves an active range of motion is a form of mobility adaptor, which involves moving a joint through a range of motion to lengthen the surrounding tissue. As muscles on one side of a joint contract, the muscles on the opposite side lengthen to allow the movement. Repetition adapts mobility.

Eccentric loading

Once you have completed the early stages of the programme and your strength has improved, your body starts to strive for further stimulus. At this point I have added some 'eccentric' loading work, so look out for the phrase midway through the plan.

The eccentric phase of a movement is the controlled positioning phase, which takes the resistance to the start point of the push or pull. So, it would be during the lowering phase of a squat, or the controlled return back to the start point in a lat pulldown. Too often we ignore this part of an exercise, but we can deal with more intensity in this part of the movement than we can in the concentric phase. Training the eccentric phase for a period of time increases our muscle growth and strength. Because we can create greater load and tension, we develop greater controlled damage to the muscle and greater adaptation. In the gym, recruit a partner to add extra load into the eccentric phase. When training alone, add more time under tension in the eccentric phase to add stimulus. The lower phase of all your exercises in this phase needs to be slow. I have gone for a three or four count here so that you will see muscle development, and also included a little kick up in the weight when you go back to normal reps.

Post-workout stretches

Once you've finished your workout, don't stop. The best time to stretch to improve flexibility is when your muscles are warm and pliable after exercise. Suggestions for stretches are on page 118.

→ Your workout rules

Be prepared: Make sure you have access to all the equipment you need, when you need it. There's nothing worse than finding your efforts are thwarted by a simple omission. Do your research and plan ahead.

Make sure weights are heavy enough: Using weights that are too light will do little to stimulate your growth hormone production, so it's essential that you select a weight that you can lift for the required rep range.

Always warm up: Within the plan are warm-up exercises and drills that are a vital component of the overall programme. Warm-up moves activate the muscles you are going to use strenuously later on. Don't skimp.

Make every exercise count: Each exercise is included for a reason – the compound exercises recruit the largest muscles in the body and the supersets with short rest periods really increase your production of HGH and testosterone.

Post workout stretch: This is really important as the best time to stretch is after a workout.

Recover well: Make sure you allow your body a day off between workouts. This is essential to allow your muscles to repair and rebuild.

Have a clean sleeping routine: Make sure you put into practice the tips in the sleep and recovery chapter. There's never been a time in your life when sleep is more important. If you struggle with sleep, start by limiting caffeine after 2pm and ban yourself from using electronic devices before going to bed.

Look after soft tissue: Your body is going to be working really hard over the next two months – you must treat it well. The soft tissue roller work exercises I've included (see page 120) are a great way to relieve tightness and to release the fascial tissue that can thicken and tighten and cause problems.

Factor Two
Recovery

Often overlooked in a fitness regimen, recovery is hugely important – particularly so as we age. Fail to factor it in and you are asking for problems

Physical exercise is just a stimulus for improving our body and it does not matter how much time we spend exercising if we do not work effectively and efficiently and we do not maximise the recovery process. I teach my clients how recovery is vital for success, but more importantly how it is crucial for a long and healthy lifestyle. Monitoring our daily patterns of sleep, stress, eating, training, moving and sitting is essential to understand what we are, what we do and how we can gradually embrace change. The recovery process, in the wider aspect of it, needs to embrace both physical recovery and mental recovery. You can read much more about the science behind recovery in Chapter 7.

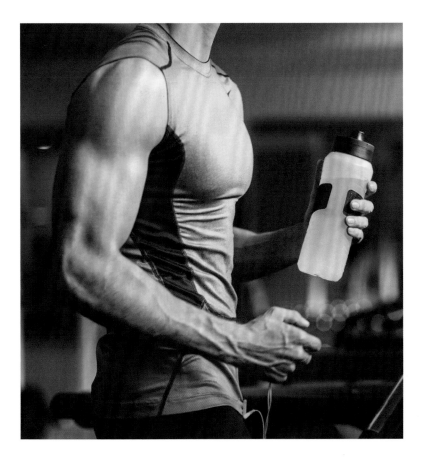

Matt Says:

It's vital to keep tabs on how well you are recovering – mentally and physically – from exercise

Factor Three
Sleep

Far too many of us fail to get enough sleep to support our lifestyles. Yet a good night's rest is paramount to our overall health

Sleep is one of the most, if not the most, important stages of recovery for any human and goes a long way to determining their capacity for longevity. Without effective sleep, we cannot function optimally and therefore we cannot train effectively, recover effectively, eat effectively or think effectively. Understanding how a client sleeps and the quality of the sleep they get is something I consider a hugely important factor in their success. It is also something that needs constant checking as it will change depending on what else is going on in their life.

It's during sleep that we produce most Human Growth Hormone (HGH) from the pituitary gland. It's also at night when sleeping that the pituitary gland signals many other responses such as the production of testosterone in the testes, adaptive responses in the adrenal glands, and repair and reset signalling to the endocrine system. All are essential for looking good, feeling good, having an abundance of energy, being able to self-heal, and enjoying life in to your late 40s, 50s and beyond. 'Sleep hygiene' strategies need to be constantly assessed and monitored as you will discover in chapter 7.

Matt Says:

It's at night, when you are sleeping, that the body rebuilds and repairs itself

Sleep and T levels

The amount of high-quality sleep we routinely achieve has a huge effect on the amount of testosterone our bodies naturally produce.

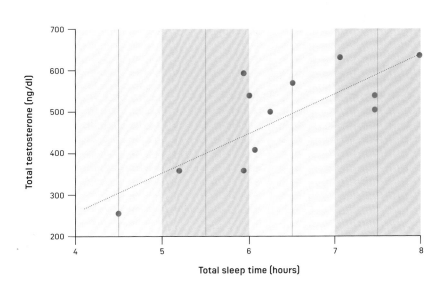

Diet

What you eat influences not only how much you weigh, but your overall health and vitality. In my plan, you will learn to eat nutritious and hormone-enhancing foods that won't leave you feeling hungry

We are asking many things from our diets as we get older. We want food that is nutrient dense and that will support our lifestyles and our activity patterns, but we also want a diet that will maximise our hormonal status and ensure us longevity. It's a lot to ask, but the eating plan I'm advocating has been tried and tested on dozens of my clients – and it works. Not only that, it is rich in flavours and variety. You certainly won't get bored and the feedback I've had from men who've tried it is that they barely remember they are on a diet plan.

Each day I've made sure there's plenty of the fibre that's essential for healthy gut flora, or microbiota, as well as a daily protein kick, essential for repairing and building those muscles that will be working so hard. I've also aimed to keep the glycaemic-low (GI) carbs to a minimum. Let's be clear, this is not a 'low carb' diet and you will not go hungry from avoiding starchy foods. However, the choice of carbs I'm recommending is from fibrous and satiating sources like brown rice, wild rice, rye breads, vegetables and legumes.

Think hormone boost

A priority is to increase all the natural nutrients that will enhance production of testosterone and HGH at the same time as increasing the natural inhibitors of the female hormone oestrogen in the body. This will

Matt Says:

A good protein intake is essential to stimulate growth hormone production

have the effect of maximising muscle growth while reducing the amount of body fat you store.

As we get older our ability to exercise as hard for as long diminishes. In middle-aged men, this is largely down to the huge reduction in the amount of testosterone produced by the body, and also the gradually decreasing levels of HGH excreted from the pituitary gland. Testosterone is 25 per cent lower at age 45 than at age 20, and the available HGH is 40 per cent lower at age 45 than it is at age 20. That's not all. From middle age onwards, a man's levels of oestrogen go up. This is what causes those much-feared fat deposits in 'female' areas of the hips and the chest.

Think protein

This is an essential aspect of your diet plan. We need to fuel the body with plenty of protein in order to stimulate HGH production. And it should come in the form of protein from foods as well as supplemented amino acids and BCAAs. But we don't want a diet that is excessively high in protein. Why? Because it strains the ageing digestive system. So rather than the 2.2-2.5g/kg body weight of protein daily for a younger man, you will be consuming somewhere in the region of 1.8g/kg body weight of protein daily, along with other nutrients that can directly influence testosterone production.

Think herbs and supplements

There are various supplements that have been shown to have excellent results when it comes to sending testosterone levels into overdrive. We are looking at D-aspartic acid (D-AA), fenugreek and oyster extract as the best researched with the best results. These nutrients, used alongside vitamins D and K,

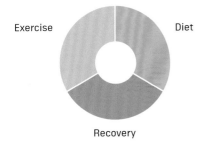

Exercise Diet

Recovery

Exercise alone wil not deliver the results for which you're searching, but the workouts will create the stimulation for the body to rebuild and repair. Combined with the correct diet, and adequate recovery, you'll access the positive changes you desire

vitamins B6 and B12, and folic acid, have shown huge improvements in male hormone production in as little as ten days.

Think fasting

Twice a week I will be asking you to fast. Fasting days are designed to reset your natural hormone trigger, to allow the natural detoxification of the body and to give your digestive system a well-deserved break

from all the hard work it does. It's easier than you might think. I advocate a 16:8 approach – a gentle form of daily intermittent fasting that sees you fast for around 16 hours and have an eating window that lasts for eight hours. Overleaf, I cover the basic how-tos regarding fasting; for more detailed insight see chapter 3, Nutrition.

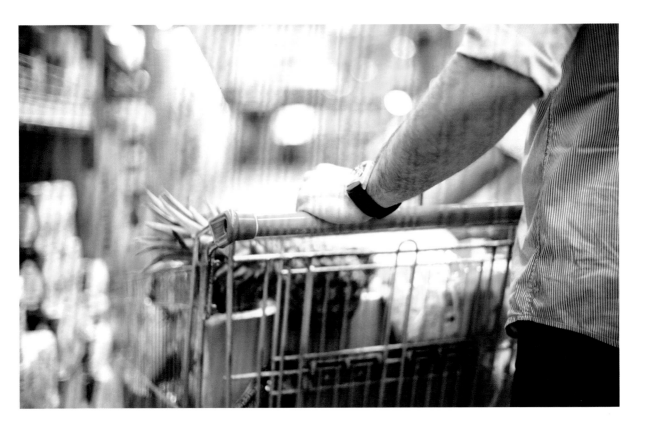

How to fast:

Start gently: If you haven't attempted anything like this before, start gradually with a 13-hour fast and an 11-hour eating window before moving slowly towards the 16:8 pattern. If you usually eat breakfast at 9am and have your last meal at 8:30pm, for example, try pushing breakfast back to 10am and bringing dinner forward to 7:30pm.

Plan ahead: Decide when your eating window will be. Pick nights and days in which you will obviously not be too exposed to temptations, commitments or distractions such as work events, parties, etc.

Choose your foods: Plan the meals you will be eating during your eating window, which should amount to around 700–800 calories.

Stay in the moment: Try to think about how you actually feel during the 16-hour period. For many people there is actually a sense of great control, calm and balance as you aren't exposed to peaks and troughs in sugar levels.

Keep it low-key: The practicality of using fasting is something that is unique to you, your routine and your environment. Because you need around 16 hours of straight fasting it is, clearly, imperative that this period is as easy to stick to as possible.

Have a night-time fast: For anybody, 16 hours can feel like a long time not eating, so for many it is easiest to schedule the fasting phase while you are asleep. For example, if you start the 16-hour fast period at around 4pm you will be breaking it 16 hours later at 8am. In effect, you are simply skipping dinner and having breakfast at around 8am in the morning, after which you will have your eight-hour period on a controlled intake (through lunch) until you resume the regular eating regime at around 4pm again.

Don't cheat: The key thing once you start the process is that you don't break or cheat it. We are looking for a specific response from the body that requires the timings, consumption and activity to be correct, so don't assume that going in with 90 per cent effort is going to be enough.

Break the fast with a workout: When your 16-hour fast period is over, you need to exercise hard at around 9am in the morning, using one of the strength training programmes at a high loading and level. It's at this point that the spike in HGH happens, encouraging cellular growth and recovery, and also increases in testosterone, not to mention the anti-ageing effects of doing the workout.

→ # What your fasting day might look like

Everyone is different and you can choose your fasting menu to suit your own personal tastes. Within the diet plan I've included a basic outline of what you should be eating that day, but really the choice is yours – just make sure those 700–800 calories are as nutrient-packed as possible. On my own fasting days, I normally have a green vegetable smoothie with avocado and 25g of protein at 10am, a kale, pear, carrot and spinach juice at noon, a 150g chicken breast with broccoli and salad and a cup of matcha tea at 2pm, a green vegetable smoothie with 25g of protein at 5pm, and a smoothie with apple, ginger, mint, lemon and water at 6pm.

→ Your Diet Rules

Success on any plan comes down to consistency and routine. Stick hard and fast to these rules, and you'll see results

Plan ahead: This is crucial. The better prepared you are, the easier it will be to stick to all aspects of your plan. Shop ahead and even cook some basic foods in advance, storing them in the fridge so that they are ready to use when you need them.

Know your regimen: Each week you have four training days when you will have a slightly higher calorie intake, one day that is non-training and non-fasting and two fasting days. Once you make yourself familiar with this regimen it will become incredibly easy to follow.

Avoid creamy sauces: This is relatively easy to do at home, but less so when you are eating out. What you also want to avoid is too much butter and oil added to foods. If in doubt when you are in a restaurant, always ask how something is cooked.

Limit alcohol: If you can avoid alcohol altogether for eight weeks, then I recommend doing that. However, if social and work commitments revolve around it, then limit yourself to two days a week when you are allowed to drink. Remember, alcohol is formed from sugar and provides empty calories that are heading nowhere but your waistline and moobs. I've seen best results from male clients who substantially cut the amount they drink.

Drink three cups of fluid first thing: Apart from on the fasting days, when you wake up, make yourself a glass of warm lemon water. Coffee with breakfast is fine. In fact, coffee has been shown to enhance the kind of effects we are after on this plan. The rules are that it should be black, ideally, or served with only a small amount of milk and definitely no sugar. If you aren't a coffee fan, try tea, again with only small amounts of milk and no sugar.

Drink two litres of water on fasting days: Fluid intake is essential, although on fasting days you do need to be strict with yourself and avoid tea, coffee, fruit juice, diet drinks and alcohol.

Don't eat every time you are hungry: Get out of the habit of grazing. Schedule your meal times and stick to them. Eat when it is time for you to eat what you have planned to eat.

Make meals colourful: If your plate of food is a vibrant array of colours and textures, it's a sure sign that it has a wide range of nutrients.

Aim for 10 portions a day: Yes, that's right, I advocate not the five daily portions of fruit and veg that the UK government recommends, but double that amount – every day (apart from when you are fasting). Don't worry, you will find it relatively easy. It's more of a habit than anything else. The bulk of these 10 portions should come from vegetables (which contain fewer natural sugars) than fruit, but the key is to get a variety. They are essential for a long, healthy life.

Make healthy eating a habit: If you create a routine that suits you, you are much more likely to stick with the principles of my eating plan. Healthy eating – like healthy living – comes down to good habits. And with our work, family and social life prone to unpredictable patterns, our diet and exercise is one thing we can control. Make it your aim that it becomes a healthy habit.

Digestive Health

Emerging science is uncovering the huge importance that a healthy gut and good digestion plays in our overall health and in the ageing process. Your diet will be primed to getting it right

It might seem the least important, but I can't emphasise enough how crucial it is to have good digestive health. Fail to address this factor and your efforts will be diluted. If you are going to maximise your training efforts, you need to have blood that is full of nutrients and cells that can produce energy. If you are to sleep well, you need to make sure that you are not going to bed with a digestive system that is under stress and having to break down food and produce gases, the by-products of poor digestion, that can cause insomnia. By becoming more conscious about the foods you eat, you can make sure your digestive system is breaking foods down quickly and passing those nutrients out through the intestinal walls into the blood stream. And all of this comes down to how and why we feed the healthy bacteria-rich environment of the gut. You will be finding out much more about how and why we must make sure that our gut bacteria and digestive enzyme levels conspire to create a stress-free digestive system in chapter 4. I can't stress enough that, even if you get everything else on this plan absolutely spot on, results will not be optimal if digestive health is off kilter.

Matt Says:

The by-products of poor digestion can cause insomnia and interfere with progress on the plan

Speed Read

→ There are five important factors of the plan: exercise, recovery, diet and nutrition, sleep and digestive health.

→ Weight training (and learning how to lift) are crucial for maximising testosterone gains.

→ Sleep is the time when we produce human growth hormone and testosterone – don't skimp on it.

→ As we age, it is hugely important to schedule in full recovery times. This enables our bodies to respond positively to the efforts we are placing on them.

→ Your diet must be varied and should not leave you feeling hungry most days.

→ Fasting is something that we will be doing twice weekly – although the approach is not extreme – and you will reap the benefits in terms of hormone production and weight maintenance.

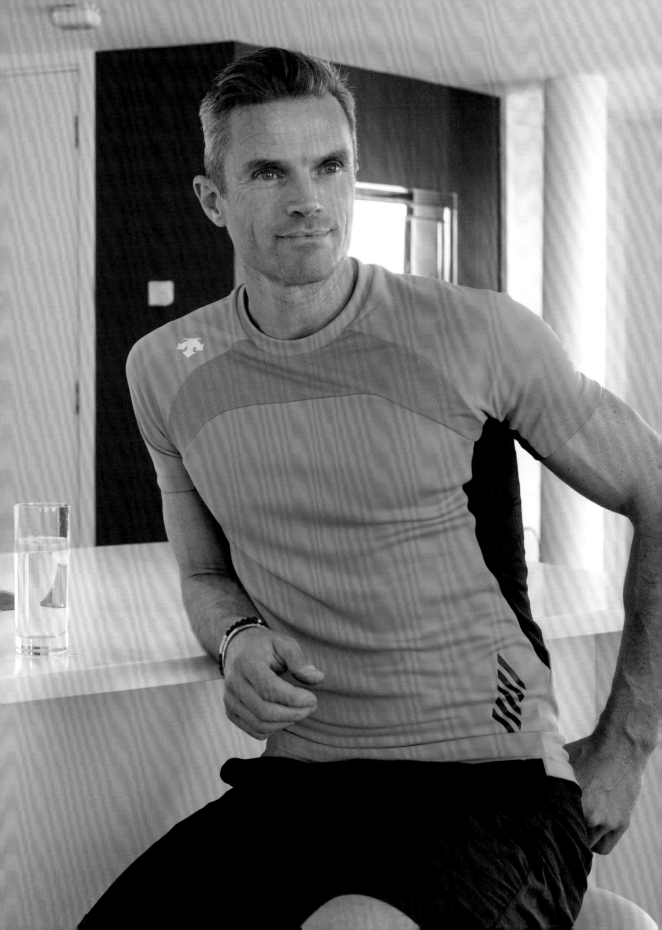

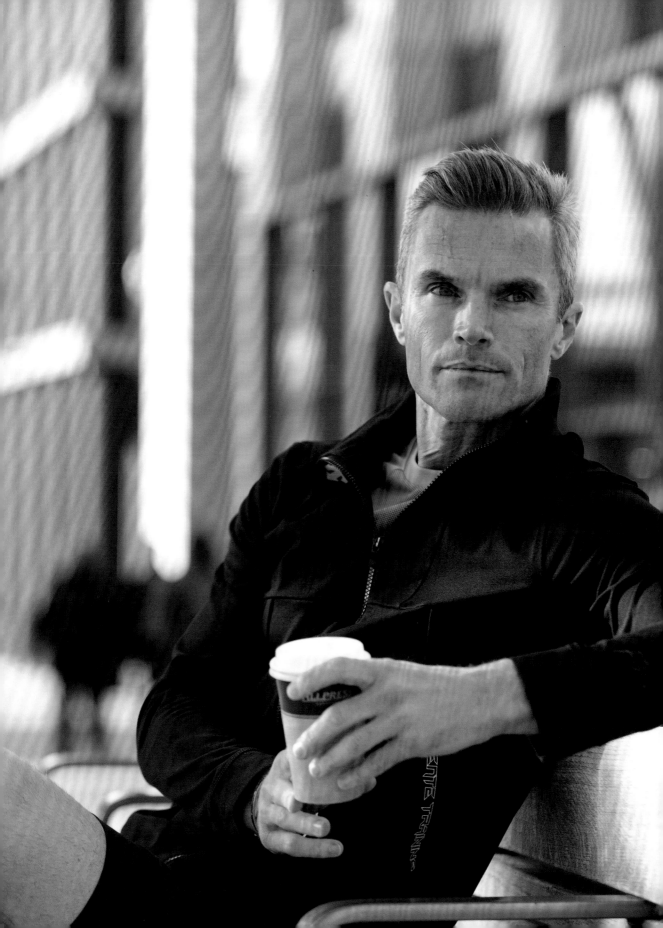

Nutrition

Transforming your shape is not possible without transforming your diet, and choosing the right food plays a crucial role in releasing testosterone and growth hormones into your system. I'm not in favour of being too draconian or evangelical about diet: food should be nutritious, but it should also be enjoyed. It is possible to have a fantastic physique while eating well every day. On this programme you should not go hungry and may find you are eating more calories than before yet with visible benefits to your physical transformation.

Diet Goals

Everyone responds to clearly set goals and I'll be outlining a few for you to aim for here. Don't worry – they are not too restrictive and you certainly won't go hungry

What we are aiming for is a diet that will help to block levels of the female hormone, oestrogen (that's the one that causes those unsightly moobs and a fat middle) and to enhance testosterone levels so that your body loses fat and builds muscle as effectively as possible. This is not as daunting as it sounds and can be achieved by eating a 'lean', balanced diet based on high quality proteins such as meat and fish, with low GI carbs. Your daily diet should feature lots of green and cruciferous vegetables, such as kale, broccoli, cauliflower and watercress, which are rich in antioxidant vitamins that help reboot energy production within your cells, and foods rich in vitamin K, a natural testosterone booster, such as eggs, Brussels sprouts, spinach, prunes and kefir.

Don't eat too little

The worst thing you can do is to starve yourself by limiting calories. Cutting healthy carbs too severely in diets can be very effective in reducing body fat but counterproductive for hormones in the long term. The reason for this is that a diet low in carbohydrates can reduce testosterone production over a long period of time. High quality natural carbohydrates help to lower cortisol (a testosterone inhibitor), support metabolism, support thyroid function and increase tryptophan (improving quality of sleep). All of these factors link into the three main influences on testosterone levels that we detailed at the beginning (see chapter 1). The role of carbohydrates should therefore not be ignored when looking to increasing testosterone levels.

Similarly, low fat diets are also detrimental to testosterone production. The body requires high-quality fats to produce hormones and therefore a lack of these will affect testosterone levels. Fat and cholesterol are the raw ingredients for testosterone and are required to transport and absorb the fat-soluble vitamins A, D, E and K; two of which (D and K) are essential for healthy testosterone levels.

You will be working hard and your body's musculature will need somewhere in the region of 2,700 calories a day to make the changes asked of it. Eating enough throughout the day also helps to keep your blood sugar stable, further enhancing the release of testosterone. Believe me, although the calorie count seems high, it is essential for repair, recovery and growth of your muscles and cellular system. Remember that our appetite hormones can be trained like anything else, so be patient and your body will soon adapt to the new regimen.

Matt Says:

Every time you shop try a new type of fruit or vegetable you haven't tried before. Keeping your ingredients interesting is really important mentally

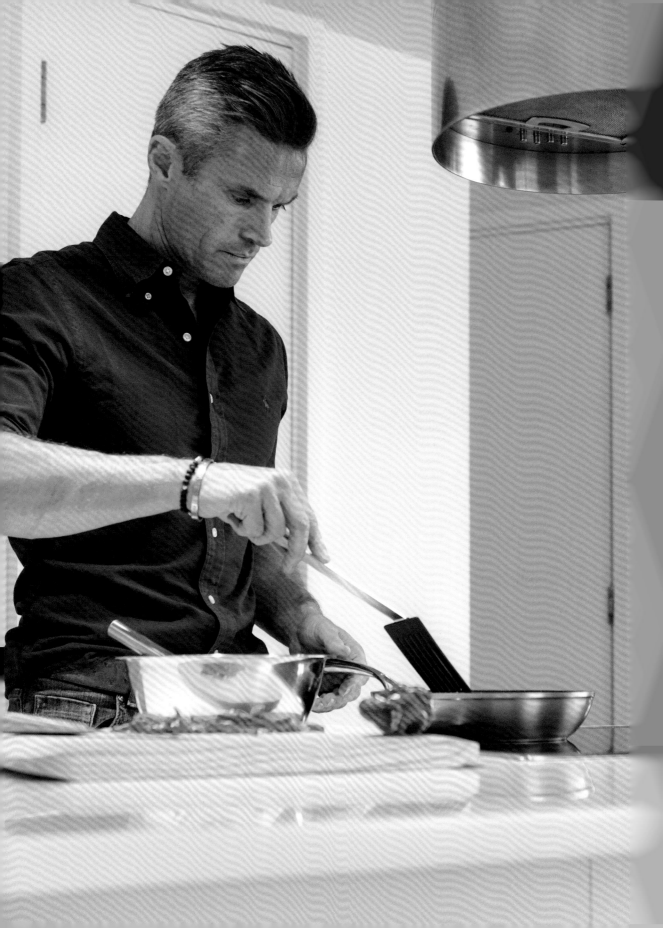

What to Avoid

Maximize the benefits of the plan by avoiding these common pitfalls

There are certain things I recommend you don't eat or drink on the programme. It may be challenging, but I'm sure you'll agree it's a good idea to avoid de-railing your own progress where you can.

Alcohol

This should be kept to an absolute minimum but preferably avoided while you are on the programme. Not only will high intakes of alcohol cause you to gain weight because of the excess calories it provides, but it is the enemy of testosterone production. Studies [1] have found that even moderate intakes of alcohol can lower blood testosterone levels by up to 6.8 per cent. Chemicals present in some alcoholic beverages include phytoestrogen and prolactin, both of which can increase oestrogen and therefore decrease testosterone production. The flowers of the hop plant used to give beer its flavour are known to be very high in phytoestrogens, the plant compounds that can mimic the action of the female sex hormone oestrogen in your body. It's complex and, as yet, unproven, but it's suggested that too much alcohol, specifically beer, might cause hormonal changes in men that increase the risk of storing belly fat.

I'm conscious that, for some people, it's socially difficult to cut out alcohol completely. But by reducing it as much as possible, you are setting yourself up for a positive hormonal equilibrium.

Sugar and processed foods

This includes anything containing unnecessary sugar, which generally means processed foods are out, as are sugary and fizzy drinks. There are important reasons for this. Sugary foods send insulin levels soaring and growth hormone and testosterone plummeting. In short, insulin not only promotes fat storage but suppresses male hormone release which is the opposite of what we are trying to achieve.

There's plenty of evidence to support the fact that you should reduce unnecessary sugar. Researchers from Massachusetts General Hospital in Boston, USA, found that a sugar shot was associated with a significant decrease in testosterone. Just 75g of sugar intake was enough to cause a sharp and significant drop in testosterone levels for up to two hours after consumption [2]. Analysing the responses of 74 men aged from 19 to 74, they noticed that ingesting sugar resulted in a 25 per cent decrease in testosterone levels, which remained suppressed for two hours. At least 10 of the 66 men with normal circulating testosterone at the start of the experiment experienced a reduction in the sex hormone levels below the low testosterone range.

We consume too much sugar and it comes mainly in the form of processed and refined foods – biscuits, cereals, cakes and ready meals – and fizzy drinks, so by cutting down on these you will drastically reduce your intake. Within the programme, you will still satisfy your sweet tooth, but with naturally occurring sugars in fruits and vegetables that are present in conjunction with valuable nutrients. And let me make a promise to you: after a couple of weeks, the changes to your body and mood will prove you don't need that sugar rush at all.

Fast Benefits

For two days a week I will be asking you to restrict your food consumption to within a scheduled 'eating window'

As discussed on page 32-33, on two days per week of the programme, you will be fasting. Don't be alarmed by the word – fasting is nowhere near as scary as it sounds. Many of my clients are wary of the prospect of going without food, but my approach is a 'gentle' 16:8 fast, that means restricting food intake to an eight-hour window and not eating for the remaining 16 hours.

Plan it carefully and you can make sure that most of those 16 hours without food are spent sleeping. What's more, the physical benefits of the approach are enormous. From research we know that, after fasting for a short but sustained period and then breaking that period with an intensive workout, we actually get a spike in human growth hormone that is three or four times the level that we might have exhibited if we hadn't.

How will it help?

There's plenty of research that has shown how men aged 40 plus who want to gain muscle, strip away some fat and benefit from a growth hormone push and raised testosterone levels respond well to this type of intermittent fasting. Studies indicate the approach helps to reduce blood lipids, blood pressure, markers of inflammation and oxidative stress in middle-aged men (and women).

Leading much of the research into the 16:8 approach is Krista Varady, Associate Professor of Kinesiology and Nutrition in the University of Illinois's College of Applied Health Sciences in the USA. In one of her trials [3], Varady looked at 23 obese volunteers who had an average age of 45. Between 10am and 6pm, the dieters could eat any type and quantity of food they liked, but for the remaining 16 hours they could only drink water or diet drinks. The study

followed the participants for 12 weeks. Compared with a control group who followed a different fasting approach, the 16:8 group consumed about 350 fewer calories, lost about 3 per cent of their body weight and saw their systolic blood pressure decrease by about 7 millimeters of mercury (mm Hg).

Intermittent fasting can also be a powerful tool in boosting your insulin sensitivity and hormonal balance. When you eat, your levels of growth hormone and testosterone drop, but during a period of fasting their production and release into the body are accelerated. By consuming all of your calories in the reduced window, you're not negatively altering your hormones throughout the whole day. Reduced levels of the hormone IGF-1 (insulin-like growth factor, a protein produced by the liver) have been noted in people who practise intermittent fasting. Since high levels of IGF-1 are believed to significantly increase the risks of colorectal and prostate cancer, you can begin to see the additional benefits.

A twice weekly fast also induces a process called autophagy where your cells remove toxins and oestrogenic – or female – chemicals. It's an approach underpinned by sound science that I urge you to try.

Matt Says:

The huge push of testosterone that follows a period of fasting is enhanced if you can train the morning after a fasting day, before eating your first meal

→ Your Hormone-enhancing Foods

Stock your cupboards with these oestrogen-inhibiting, testosterone-boosting foods to ensure you are starting from the best possible point:

Omega-3 Fats: Sardines, walnuts, salmon and mackerel are all great sources of omega-3 essential fatty acids, which are known to help reduce stress and inflammation in the body and act as a powerful anti-inflammatory. Testosterone is what we refer to as an anabolic hormone, which means that it promotes growth and repair within the body, and is released most effectively in a low-stress environment. So, by lowering inflammation and stress, omega-3s help testosterone production to increase. Added to that is the effect these important fats have on the hormone cortisol, which is released when the body experiences stress. Cortisol, a catabolic hormone, counteracts the role of testosterone, promoting the breakdown of muscles and inflammation. Testosterone production is one of the hormones that is inhibited at this time. Getting enough omega-3 in your diet is crucial, but I would also recommend a supplement to support the diet.

Honey: It contains small amounts of the mineral boron and also the flavonoid chrysin that has been found to block the conversion of male hormones into oestrogens.

Eggs: High in protein and healthy fats, eggs also contain vitamin D, a known growth hormone stimulant.

Zinc: Shellfish, crab, lobster, oysters, beef, mussels, pumpkin seeds, spinach and cashew nuts are all great sources of this mineral which acts as an aromatase inhibitor, meaning that it blocks oestrogen receptor sites. The result is that it helps to reduce the amount of testosterone that is converted into oestrogen leading to higher overall levels of testosterone in the body.

Mushrooms: Studies have shown that the phytochemicals in mushrooms can block an enzyme called aromatase from producing oestrogen. And you don't need to spend a fortune on exotic varieties – plain white button mushrooms have been shown to have an effect. Researchers at Beckman Research Institute showed how an extract prepared from white button mushrooms decreased the activity of the aromatase enzyme and lowered oestrogen levels in a dose-dependent manner (i.e. the more eaten, the greater the effect) [4]. Another study found that eating white button mushrooms in combination with drinking green tea had a 'statistically significant' effect on inhibiting aromatase enzyme activity [5]. Varieties such as shiitake, chanterelle and portobello are thought to be effective too.

Selenium: Foods rich in this mineral boost testosterone production. Crab, liver and Brazil nuts are good sources.

Cruciferous vegetables: Broccoli, kale, Brussels sprouts, watercress, bok choy and cauliflower are all great vegetables to include in your daily diet. They contain a compound called indole-3-carbinol that may reduce levels of oestrogen and promote healthier levels of testosterone in men's bodies. Indoles work by converting excess oestrogen into a safer form, shown to reduce the risk of prostate cancer. That, in turn, can help reduce oestrogen's inhibitory effect on testosterone production.

Vitamin K: This vitamin is a potent testosterone booster that has clinical trials to prove its effectiveness. You will find it in eggs, kale, Brussels sprouts, broccoli, prunes and kefir.

Antioxidants: These help to boost energy levels in your cells. Include cruciferous vegetables (kale, bok choy, cauliflower, watercress), matcha green tea, cordyceps mushrooms, turmeric and chillies in your diet.

Amino acids: Leucine is among the most important amino acid for enhancing male hormones. You'll find it in cheese, soybeans, beef, chicken, pork, nuts, seeds, fish and seafood.

Cholesterol: It has had a lot of bad press, but it is very important to understand that dietary cholesterol rarely negatively affects blood cholesterol levels. Cholesterol is made by every cell in the body and is incredibly important to overall health. What's more, it's an essential ingredient for hormone production and plays an important role in the synthesis of testosterone. By avoiding foods that have a high cholesterol level, you could be harming your hormone balance and health. Eggs, chicken, butter, beans, fatty fish, flax seeds and olive oil all help to increase the body's levels of HDL ('good' cholesterol), so make sure you include them.

Carrots and sweet potatoes: Rich in beta-carotene and chemically-related carotenoid compounds, these brightly coloured vegetables may help to reduce the growth of oestrogen receptors in the body.

Oats and wholegrains: These foods are rich in fibre that will aid digestion and promote healthy gut bacteria. They may also help to block oestrogens.

Signs of low testosterone

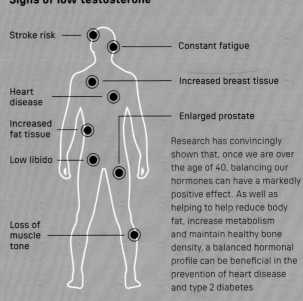

Stroke risk

Constant fatigue

Increased breast tissue

Heart disease

Enlarged prostate

Increased fat tissue

Low libido

Loss of muscle tone

Research has convincingly shown that, once we are over the age of 40, balancing our hormones can have a markedly positive effect. As well as helping to help reduce body fat, increase metabolism and maintain healthy bone density, a balanced hormonal profile can be beneficial in the prevention of heart disease and type 2 diabetes

Supplements to Consider

There is no magic potion for improved fitness and health, but sometimes a supplement can provide the edge you need to inch closer to your goals. Below are some that might help to enhance your hormonal balance

Don't think you can find anything in a bottle or powder that will replace the need for hard work. No supplement will ever replace a good exercise programme and a healthy diet. However, as we age there are supplements that can make it easier for men to realise the goal of boosting hormone production.

My team has done lots of research into this area and we are convinced that some herbs and naturally derived products are a boost to this 8-week programme.

D-aspartic acid: An amino acid that plays a role in making and releasing hormones in the body, it is available in capsule form. It increases the release of brain hormones that ultimately result in testosterone production and also plays a role in increasing testosterone production and release in the testicles.

Oyster body extract: This is a natural taurine, zinc and micro-nutrient complex, containing natural trace minerals, vitamins, omega oils and amino acids. Oyster extract is an all-natural way to help increase your testosterone levels due to the high level of zinc it is made up of. It also reportedly helps enhance libido and sexual performance in men.

Fenugreek: This herb boosts libido and stimulates testosterone levels. It also increases insulin release, which can help increase muscle mass after weight training

Gamma aminobutyric acid (or GABA): Available as a capsule, it helps stimulate HGH release.

Mucuna pruriens: An extract of an Indian creeping vine that is renowned for promoting HGH production. It comes in powder, supplement or tincture form.

Maca root: Rich in essential minerals, selenium, calcium, magnesium and iron, it also contains an assortment of vitamins including C, E, B1 (thiamine) and B2 (riboflavin) as well as 20 different fatty acids and 19 amino acids and polysaccharides which support healthy energy levels. Comes in powder or capsule form and can be added to smoothies.

Resveratrol Pro Q10: Contains concentrated levels of polyphenols, trans-resveratrol from red grape skin, the root of the Japanese Knotweed plant and the naturally derived nutrient Coenzyme Q10. Both trans-resveratrol and Co-Q10 are rapidly metabolised and eliminated by the body. Reputedly good for preventing release of the female hormone oestrogen, it comes in capsule and tablet form.

Matt Says:

Supplement for success. For optimal success on my programme I cannot encourage you enough to add in the extra testosterone boosting supplements, high potency anti-oxidants, protein shakes and snacks, BCAAs and good quality fish oils that will help you reach your target goals

Stinging nettle root: Good for preventing release of the female hormone oestrogen. Available as a tea or a powder.

Branched-chain amino acids (or BCAAs): Taking branched-chain amino acids before a workout is a great way to maximise hormone release. Available as a powder or in capsule form.

L-glutamine: This is what is referred to as a conditionally essential amino acid. We can synthesise L-glutamine from our muscles, but as we get older and if we are training hard, the likelihood is you will not be producing enough. Supplementing with L-glutamine has been shown to reduce free radical and toxin build-up, help speedy recovery from exercise, reduce the feeling of fatigue, increase muscle adaptation to exercise and lead to a stronger cardio response. Available as a capsule or tablet.

Ashwagandha: A herb that improves anxiety, depression and insomnia, and increases overall productivity.

Water hyssop: This herb works on your nervous system. It improves your memory, judgment and reasoning, keeping you relaxed but alert at the same time.

Cordyceps sinensis: Derived from mushrooms, this herbal supplement is an immune booster and contains chemical constituents like ergosterol, alpha aminoisobutyric acid and a number of peptides that are responsible for its unique stress-busting abilities. You can consume the mushroom itself, but extracts are available in powder or capsule form.

Holy basil: Helps control blood sugar, blood pressure and stress hormone levels, such as of adrenaline and glucagon, maintaining the body equilibrium. Available as a tincture, tablet or capsule.

Rhodiola rosea: Handles symptoms from chronic stress like imperfect work performance, sleep difficulties, poor appetite, irritability, headaches and fatigue. Available as a tincture, tablet or capsule.

Vitamin D: Much has been written and researched about this vitamin in recent years and we know that the 'sunshine vitamin', so called because it is derived from sunlight, is vital for healthy bones and teeth. More interestingly for men of our age is the need for good levels of vitamin D to support the immune system and insulin control. For these reasons it's helpful in diabetes prevention and offsetting many of the diseases that become more common as we get older. Widely available as a capsule or tablet.

What about T-Box?

Having researched the nutrients needed to combat ageing after the age of 40, my team of nutritionists has come up with a complete programme of supplements – called T-Box – that will help to boost testosterone and vitality and improve your training results. It's a potent mix of vitamins, minerals and herbs that combine to provide the ultimate wellness prescription. It includes many of the lesser known, but hugely beneficial, supplements listed in this chapter that might prove tricky to track down, including Japanese knotweed, pine bark extract and maca powder alongside others such as vitamins D and K. I take it myself and can testify that it works. But don't just take my word for it. Dozens of clients have found their bodies and lives improved after using it. More information about T-Box is available on my website.

Workout Nutrition

Deciding what and when to eat before and after a workout can seem like a minefield of choices. In fact, the rules are surprisingly simple

Before you exercise

Your goal is to build muscle and to do that your body must be primed and in an anabolic state (ready to build and repair) before you start exercising. The steps below are nutritional protocols to follow before any training session as they will help you keep testosterone high for as long as possible:

Eat good quality protein: A pre-workout protein meal around 30 minutes before you hit the gym will increase the protein balance of your body

and push it into an anabolic state, switching on the muscle building process. There are many ways you can get this pre-workout protein, but among my favourites are plain Greek yoghurt with berries and granola, a banana with nut butter and honey, an apple with almond butter and raisins or a protein-rich smoothie. If you struggle to eat anything before exercising, a supplement of BCAAs (branched-chain amino acids) is worth considering. Made up of the three essential amino acids the body requires to switch on the muscle building process, a BCAA supplement will include the important amino acid leucine. You need 2.5-3g of leucine to elicit the required anabolic effect, so ensure the supplement you purchase has the adequate amount.

Carbohydrates: Although carbohydrates don't alter the muscle building response, carb-rich foods might help to reduce the rate of muscle breakdown by reducing the level of cortisol in the body. As we know, cortisol is a stress hormone and the enemy of testosterone production. By reducing cortisol, you ensure a positive impact on testosterone levels when you exercise.

Carbohydrates with protein: Research has shown that when protein and carbohydrates are consumed together they have a much greater impact on muscle building than when taken alone. A meal or snack that provides your body with both protein and carbohydrates will increase anabolic hormones such as testosterone and help reduce stress, creating the ideal environment for growth.

→ **Store cupboard essentials**

The diet you will be following is specifically designed to be both nutritious and widely available. However, it is helpful to prepare in advance and make sure that you have the following items ready to use in your cupboard or fridge.

→ dried chillies
→ Tabasco® sauce
→ porridge oats
→ granola
→ zatar
→ almonds
→ raisins
→ whey powder
→ rye crispbreads
→ chickpeas
→ kidney beans

After exercise

Your post-workout nutrition choices can either promote repair and recovery or potentially inhibit it. Once you have exercised, your muscles are in a state of absorption and need nutrients to repair the muscle fibres that have been damaged during the session. Your body adapts by repairing damaged muscle fibres or building more as a result of training stimulus and adequate nutritional influences. To aid this process, you need to supply nutrients that will support the anabolic response that exercise creates, maximising your growth and repair.

Carbohydrates and protein: Again, this combo is a tour de force. Research has shown that when taken within 1-3 hours post-resistance training they can increase the muscle response by 400 per cent.

Whey to go: The best protein to consumer post-workout is whey. It is derived from milk and contains high levels of the essential amino acids, which are readily digested, absorbed and retained by the body for muscle repair. There's also evidence it may enhance immune function. It is rapidly digested and quickly available to the body. The amino acids it provides drive up protein balance, pushing the body into an anabolic state. That means anabolic hormones, such as testosterone, can work effectively to repair and grow new stronger muscle fibres. I find adding it to shakes is one of the best ways to include whey protein in my diet.

High GI carbohydrates: Here we are talking about white pasta, potatoes and bread. These are best consumed post-workout, when muscles are super absorptive. Your muscles are depleted of glycogen as a result of training and the glucose in these carbs will be used for repair and not stored for fat. Another reason that carbohydrates are important at this time is because of the insulin response the high GI carbs will induce. Insulin decreases cortisol levels and allows hormones such as testosterone to dominate. Insulin will also help drive other nutrients such as protein into the muscle, helping with the recovery process.

Matt Says:

A cup of coffee is a great pre-workout stimulant. It lifts your adrenalin levels and you can perform better in your workout and push yourself harder

Speed Read

→ **Plan ahead:** Schedule your workouts and fasting days so that you know what to expect.

→ **Fasting days:** Try to eat your meals within an eight to nine-hour window.

→ **Post-fast:** Try to work out first thing the next day, while still in a fasted state. If you can do this a couple of times a week, it will ensure a huge push of testosterone and growth hormones.

→ **Take BCAAs:** Taking branched-chain amino acids before a workout is a great way to maximise hormone release.

→ **Pack in the veg:** Keep protein and veg intake high on your training days.

→ **Reserve carbs:** On training days add in carbohydrates to your post-workout meals, making sure they are low GI carbs whenever possible, such as sweet potato, quinoa, lentils, etc.

→ **Post-workout feast:** On hard training days try to make sure your biggest meal comes straight after your workout session. If that's breakfast, make it a substantial one.

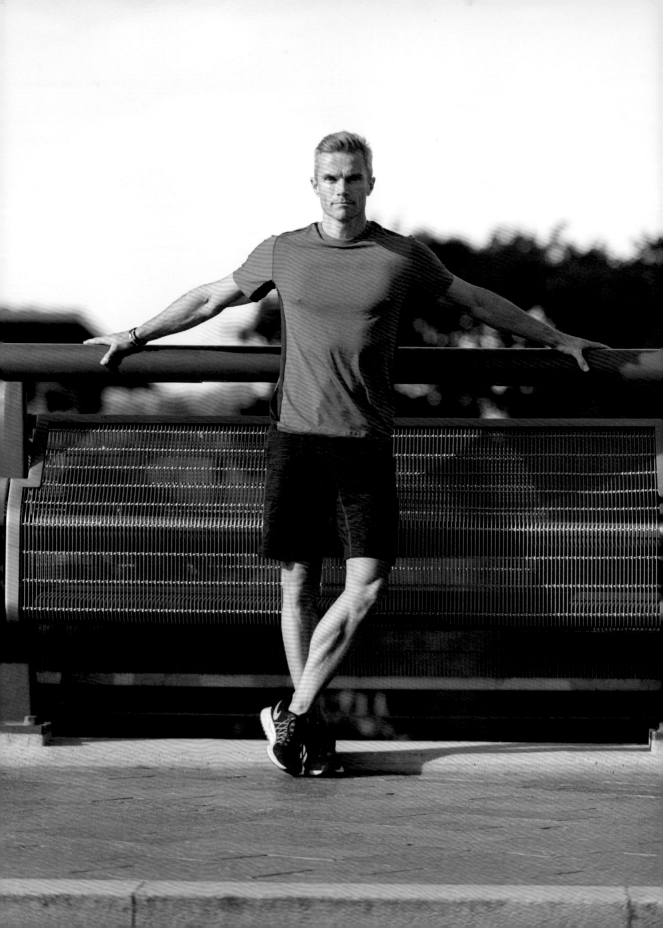

Processed Foods

Ready-made, manufactured and refined foods are often the enemy of good digestion. Best to go fresh when you can

Food that has been highly processed is food that has almost certainly seen its nutrient profile slashed. If it contained fibre in the first place, the chances are it will have been removed through milling, refining and excessive manufacturing processes. What remains are ingredients that are refined, isolated nutrients that don't resemble the whole foods they came from.

It's not only the lack of fibre and nutrients that matters to health, though. Processed food makes your digestive system slovenly. Developed to be easily consumed, these foods by their very nature take less energy to eat and digest than whole foods. We can devour more of them in a shorter amount of time (more calories in) and we burn half as many calories digesting and metabolising processed foods compared to whole foods. This is partly down to the fact that they require less chewing. When food remains in the mouth, our tongues become adept at recognising its flavours, sending messages to the brain to release the necessary digestive juices and prompting us to chew. Chewing and digesting food also fills you up. Processed foods also pass more quickly through the digestive system, so the upshot is that you're likely to feel hungry more quickly.

In his studies on twins at King's College London, Professor Spector discovered [5] that the siblings who were frailer in old age had higher levels of some microbes, including *Eubacterium dolichum*, shown in other studies to increase in unhealthy, highly processed diets. Changing your diet and lifestyle, he concluded, might be an easy way to encourage healthy ageing and digestion.

By limiting your intake of refined and processed foods, you will not only hike up your nutrient intake, but benefit your gut flora by providing more fibre and ease the strain on your digestion in the process.

Matt Says:

Eating highly refined and processed foods makes your digestive system lazy

Speed Read

→ Digestive efficiency dwindles with age so it is important that we make it a priority.

→ Our gut health is determined by the status of our microbiota, the vast ecosystem of beneficial bacteria and fungi that inhabit our gut lining.

→ Diet and exercise are key to maintaining healthy digestion, but so is stress reduction.

→ Make sure you consume enough fibre. Most men don't. Yet a high fibre diet is among the most effective steps you can take for a flourishing microbiota and good digestion.

→ A healthy digestive system means a healthy production of male hormones such as HGH and testosterone.

→ Studies have shown that people with the healthiest guts can defy ageing most successfully. They live longer and healthier lives.

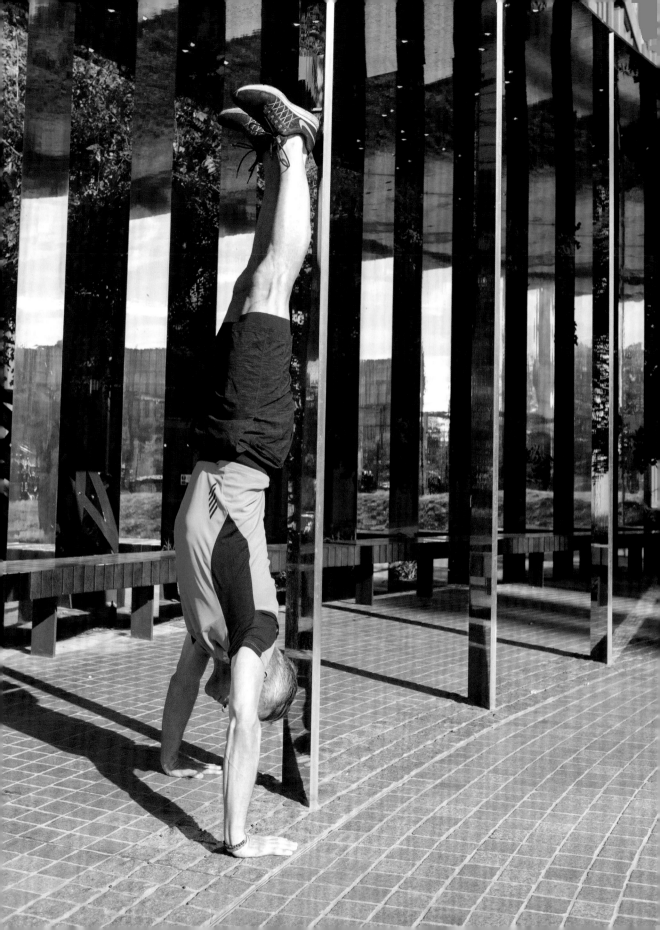

Spinal
Health

Looking after diet and exercise slow the ageing clock, but there is another aspect of your wellbeing that deserves attention: your spinal health. For decades, issues relating to back health were considered in isolation, with back pain treated as a standalone issue. But a growing number of experts around the world are convinced that spinal health deserves more attention as, if it's allowed to deteriorate, it threatens to prove our undoing.

A Healthy Spine

Our spines are the support system for our bodies and are involved in every physical movement we make. Ignore the health of your spine at your peril

So convinced am I that spinal health is key to successful ageing, I now place huge emphasis on it with my clients. And I want to do the same with you. Our spines are so much more than a simple bony structure to keep us upright and in good posture. They are integral to breathing and to every movement we make. The spinal column is made of 33 individual bones stacked one on top of the other that allows you to stand upright, bend, and twist, while protecting the spinal cord from injury.

A healthy spine is a complex network of strong muscles and bones, flexible tendons and ligaments, and sensitive nerves. But a poorly conditioned spine will impact our digestion, our ability to exercise and our mood. As breathing patterns are hampered, so supplies of oxygen to all parts of the body – the brain included – will deteriorate. Our concentration and focus, our appearance and our ability to absorb nutrients are all affected by the state of our spine. And when this spinal area is affected by strain, injury or disease, the result can be chronic and sometimes catastrophic pain.

Up to 9 million people in the UK are estimated to suffer with back pain and one in seven GP appointments is for muscle and nerve problems, most of which occur in the back. It costs the UK economy an estimated £37 million daily, with the Labour Force Survey estimating that 2.8 million working days are lost due to back problems [1].

Most fashionable back treatments are at best useless and at worst harmful with pointless (and expensive) scans, drugs, surgery and injections being prescribed to millions desperate to seek relief from their suffering. Back belts and orthotics used to correct posture were found to be almost completely ineffective by researchers [2] and educational programmes had almost zero effect. Most people who employed such methods were highly likely to experience more back pain within months.

A word of caution (as with any chronic complaint): if your back pain is either very acute or severe and long term, seek medical advice before embarking on any exercise regimen. Beyond that, the sky is the limit. What most harms our spines are lack of activity and obesity, and one of the most effective treatments is an appropriate diet and exercise programme.

What does a healthy spine look like?

Look at a healthy adult spine from a sideways-on position and it has a natural S-shaped curve. The neck (cervical) and low back (lumbar) regions have a slight concave curve, and the mid-back (thoracic) and base of the spine (sacral) regions have a gentle convex curve. At its best, this naturally curved structure works like a coiled spring to absorb shock, maintain balance, and allow a full range of movement in all directions. It's maintained by strong, well-conditioned muscles and enhanced by good lifestyle habits.

Matt Says:

An unhealthy spine triggers unwanted hormonal and metabolic changes

What makes our spines unhealthy?

Most people suffer an episode of low back pain at some point in middle age and underlying causes are often musculoskeletal, linked to damage of ligaments, joints and muscles around the spine. For some, the problem has its roots in wear and tear; this is particularly true of people who have played contact sports that may have caused damage to joints and the spine. Only one per cent of back pain cases are linked to serious disease such as an infection or cancer. Back pain recurs with distressing frequency – once you've experienced it, there's a 75 per cent chance you will have another debilitating episode within a year [1].

Through inactive lifestyles – too much time sitting down and too little exercise – people are less able to tolerate the twisting, turning and loading for which their backs were designed. We have reached a point where too many people are wary about doing anything that might directly stress their spine – and that is a recipe for disaster. In order to improve the health of our spines, we need to embark on a nutrition and exercise programme that will restore and strengthen them. And that is precisely what is outlined in this book. You will discover, in this chapter, that much of what we think we know about our spinal health is wrong.

The hormone connection

When your spine is in an unhealthy state, it brings about a cocktail of changes that can send your hormonal and metabolic status into decline. Think about it: if you are in discomfort or pain because you can't move freely, you restrict the amount of movement you do. That means that, as you age, your loss of muscle mass increases, your bone and muscle strength declines and, as a consequence, your body's production of hormones and your metabolism deteriorate. As your posture becomes more hunched, your digestion, and absorption of nutrients, will be affected and you will even breathe less effectively. Movement is key to so many of the body's functions and if you are moving less, it will exacerbate this cascade of side-effects.

According to a Labour Force survey, every year approximately **2.8 million days of work** are lost due to back, neck and muscle problems. This costs the UK economy **£37 million pounds a day**

How to Improve your Spinal Health

Thankfully, there is much we can do to strengthen and mobilise our spines, thereby boosting their health and efficiency. However, it can take a leap of faith as the steps are not always obvious

Strength matters. If you have a bad back, the chances are you have avoided weight training for fear of making it worse. The vast majority of people believe that bending to lift anything – from a heavy shopping bag to a bag of soil or sand – is harmful to a back that is in any way compromised. An Opinium survey of 2,005 adults across the UK that was commissioned by the Chartered Society of Physiotherapy [3] to investigate back pain myths revealed that 65 per cent of those questioned said they would avoid weight training for fear of it worsening their back pain. The facts paint a different picture.

Our spines are incredibly structurally strong. They are made to withstand loading and twisting, actions that are essential for strengthening all human tissue. When back pain occurs as a consequence of lifting something – heavy or otherwise – it is not the movement or the weight of the object that is the catalyst for pain, but the fact that your spine is too weak to support the action. And while weight training for back benefits seems counterintuitive, spinal experts and physiotherapists say it's one of the best things you can do. Done correctly, heavy lifting will absolutely not do any damage to your back. In fact, strengthening the muscles around it with resistance exercise is now considered more helpful than harmful for most people.

Among the first to shed light on how weights might be helpful were researchers at the University of Alberta, Canada. A decade ago they reported [4] that people who used weights to ease their lower back pain were ultimately better off than those who chose other forms of exercise. Participants in the trial, all of whom had chronic back ache, showed a 60 per cent improvement in pain and function when they took part in a 16-week exercise programme involving resistance training with dumbbells, barbells and other load-bearing exercise equipment. In contrast, volunteers who chose aerobic training like jogging or walking on a treadmill or using an elliptical trainer at the gym experienced only a 12 per cent improvement in their pain.

Since then, the continuing research has been convincing. Work [5] carried out on elite rowers, a group prone to back problems, by Fiona Wilson, Associate Professor of Physiotherapy at Trinity College Dublin, Ireland, has shown that backs strengthened through appropriate conditioning programmes are much less susceptible to pain and problems. Weight training works.

What if your back is sore after you have exercised? Soreness should not be considered the same as pain. A post-workout soreness is likely to occur with the muscles of the back just as it will in the muscles of your arms and legs after doing weights. What I am not advocating here is diving in with exceptionally heavy weights from the offset. Any exercise programme must be progressive and develop strength in a controlled way.

Bending and twisting

Another longstanding misconception is that you shouldn't bend or twist if you have back issues. If you feel discomfort when you bend to pick something up, it is more likely because you haven't performed that kind of movement properly in a bid to protect your back from pain. But to keep the back mobile and healthy, it is vital that you move it in all directions, however uncomfortable it is at the start. It's important to start gradually and not launch into

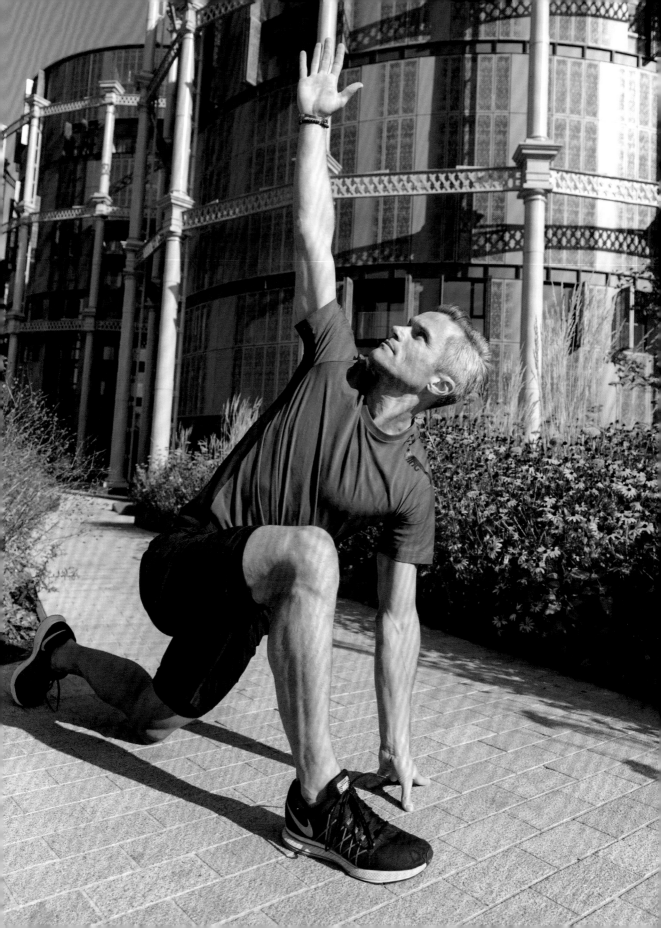

excessive bending and twisting on day one. Do a little more bending each day.

Meditation

Overcoming pain through the power of your own mind has been shown to be a powerful tool in back pain prevention. Back pain sufferers who took part in a study [6] at John Hopkins University's School of Medicine in the USA were assigned to one of two therapies – meditation or cognitive behaviour therapy – for six months. By the end of the trial, the volunteers who had been meditating found it easier to perform tasks they had previously found tricky, such as getting out of a chair, putting on socks and going upstairs. They were also less irritable and less likely to take time off work because of their bad back.

Standing up

Sitting is widely held up as the modern-day enemy of the back. As many as 65 per cent of Britons spend eight to 10 hours sitting on week days, with many sitting for eight hours even on weekends and this lack of movement is certainly one of the biggest risk factors for heart disease, stroke and diabetes. However, there are ways to make sitting less harmful to the back. At work, make sure your chair has a firm back support for your lower and middle back, and your feet can easily be placed on the floor. If you've been sitting for close to an hour, stand up and walk around. And vary the positions of the body throughout the day. Standing desks are an option, but make sure they are offer variable height options. To go from sitting all day to standing all day at a desk would be bad news for your back. Spend some time standing, some sitting, some walking, some slouching. It's about getting more movement in all directions for a healthy spine.

Vary your exercise

As I've explained, strength and weight training are essential for a healthy spine, but are any exercises better than others? Researchers at the University of Wisconsin, evaluated exercises targeting five back and shoulder muscles – the middle trapezius, lower trapezius, latissiumus dorsi, infraspinatus and erector spinae – to find out which moves were most effective when it came to strength gains. It was a small trial [7] involving 19 men, each of whom had electrodes placed on muscles so that electromyography (EMG) measurements could determine how fully they were engaged during an exercise. Results showed that no single move was effective in best recruiting all muscles in the upper and lower back. According to the exercise and sport scientists who lead the investigation, a combination of most of the exercises studied is the best bet for developing strength, but it's important to include a range of exercises that activate the back and shoulder muscle groups and also recruit other muscles to a reasonable degree.

Pick up your walking pace

Stuart McGill, Professor of Spine Biomechanics at the University of Waterloo in Canada and the author of over 400 published clinical papers on spine health, is widely regarded as the world's leading expert on back problems. And his number one tip for improving spine health and mobility is to walk more quickly on a daily basis [8]. Too many back-pain sufferers make the mistake of ambling along at a leisurely pace in the belief power-walking would exacerbate their problems and then wonder why they feel worse when they finish. That has the effect of loading the spine. With each step we take, our legs are lifted and swung in a way that produces gentle muscular contractions that prevent the pelvis from sinking. "Elastic tissues in the back reduce the amount of muscular effort needed and effectively 'unload' the spine with every stride," explains McGill. The faster you walk and the more you swing your arms – keeping your head up promotes a better arm action – the better the outcome for your back, although you should never walk 'through pain'. If your back hurts as you pick up speed, you need to progress at a steadier pace.

Stretching

A lot of people think stretching and flexibility are the sole answer for good spinal health. This is partly because some stretching moves offer temporary

→ Nutrients for a healthy spine

A healthy spine is dependent not just on movement, but on good nutrition. This is a much neglected aspect of back care and one that I am keen to address. Make sure you include the following in your diet to keep your spine mobile and strong:

Magnesium
Where found: Green leafy vegetables, fish, beans, seeds, nuts, whole grains, yogurt, avocados, bananas and dark chocolate (70% cocoa or higher).

Why needed: It's a key mineral in the structure of the bone matrix and required for more than 300 biochemical reactions in the body. If blood magnesium levels drop, magnesium will be leeched from the bones, resulting in lower bone density and potentially more back problems.

Vitamin D3
Where found: Oily fish, liver (or cod liver oil) and egg yolks.

Why needed: It aids the body's absorption of bone-building calcium, which is crucial for the development of a healthy spine.

Vitamin K1 and K2
Where found: Vitamin K1 – in green leafy vegetables such as spinach, kale, and broccoli – is the plant form of vitamin K, which is converted to vitamin K2 – found in meats, cheeses, egg yolks, and other dairy products – by healthy digestive bacteria.

Why needed: The combination of vitamin K2 and calcium works to help bones in the spine and throughout the body stay strong and healthy.

pain relief when you do them. Let me explain: when you bend the spine to stretch – as you might when touching the toes or pulling knees to the chest while lying on the floor – it triggers a neurological response called the 'stretch reflex' that leads to pain relief for about 15 minutes. However, it's not actually getting to the root of the problem. A rounded fitness regimen, such as the one I advocate in this book, is far more effective at improving all-round spinal health. What you'll find as you progress through the 8-week programme is that good nutrition and improved strength and mobility will improve all sorts of side effects that people assume are the result of back pain, including tightness in hamstrings and other muscles that often diminishes as you become stronger and fitter.

Speed Read

→ Your spine health is important not just for your posture – it can also affect your fitness, metabolism and your hormone levels.

→ Back pain is exacerbated by inactivity and weight gain.

→ Strength training – even that involving weights – is crucial for spinal conditioning.

→ Any sort of movement and activity – including bending, twisting and lifting – will help your back.

→ Good nutrition can help improve spinal health. It's important to include a range of nutrients, but particularly those that are involved in bone-building.

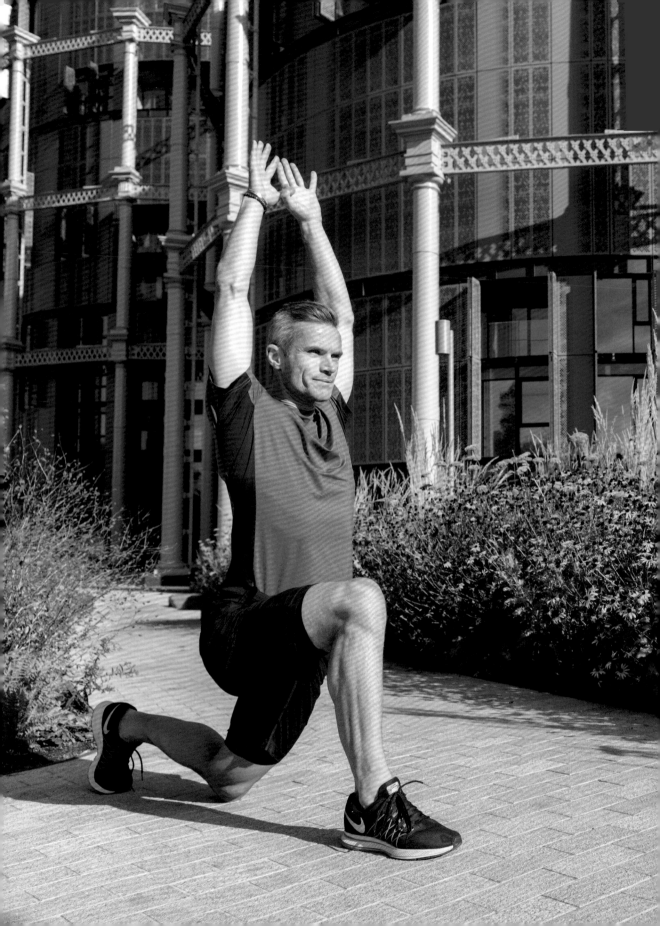

Sex and Lifestyle

Ageing has a huge effect on your hormone levels, but, as you now know, you can stem the decline of testosterone and HGH to some extent through diet and exercise. However, your hormone levels also rise and fall – both long and short term – in response to a huge number of other lifestyle factors, so these too must be brought into the equation.

Hormones and Daily Life

Diminishing hormones can affect and exacerbate everything from stress levels and sex drive to how we breathe and how successful we are at work. There are lots of ways we can redress these side-effects, however...

There are many examples of how our daily habits can cause hormones to wax and wane. Gaining too much weight causes testosterone levels to plummet – but losing 10 per cent of excess body fat can increase your testosterone count by 100 points. Drinking a few beers every so often won't make too much of a difference to your hormones (although I do advise you cut it out for maximum effect on this 8-week programme), but chronic alcohol abuse damages the liver and severely thwarts the production of testosterone. Even being left in charge of our own young children for a few hours can cause testosterone levels to drop, a study reported [1].

So let's look at how you live your life and in what ways you might be able to bring about positive changes that can prevent a steep hormonal decline.

The chemistry of stress

What contributes to stress varies hugely among individuals. It differs according to our environment and our genetics, our age and our life experiences so that what is stressful for you and I might not be for someone else. Yet an increasing number of us are prone to feeling overwhelmed. The Mental Health Foundation's 2018 report [2], the largest study of its kind, found that a staggering 74 per cent of people in the UK said they had been so stressed that they felt unable to cope.

When we encounter stress, our body responds in a number of ways, one being the stimulation of hormones that trigger the 'fight or flight' response. In sudden confrontational situations – a marital spat, a heated debate or a ticking off from your boss – the body might respond by raising levels of testosterone, a hormone that is known to induce feelings of self-confidence and aggression. This is an appropriate or even beneficial response because it helps see us through the time of tension. So, some stress, in the right quantity, is a very normal response - a natural product of our evolution.

However, the lingering anxiety caused by divorce or separation, the death of a loved one, losing a job and unexpected money problems – our most highly ranked stressors [3] – are the kind of things that set us on a path towards chronic stress. For many, a 40-hour week has become a 24/7 ordeal resulting in a perpetual state of hyper arousal. And when stress becomes this chronic or excessive – as many of us experience in our daily lives – the outcome for hormones is rarely positive. As we know, stress produces the hormone cortisol which is known to inhibit testosterone production in men. In high levels, cortisol can degrade muscle tissue and turn off your libido.

There are other reasons this is bad news. Too much cortisol lingering around in the system will interfere with the body's natural ability to heal by hampering the immune system, stripping away bone density and increasing weight gain, blood pressure and cholesterol. Prolonged exposure to cortisol has a major age-accelerating effect on the body. Can you imagine how a cortisol-flooded, stressed-

Matt Says:

Stress produces the hormone cortisol which is known to prevent testosterone production

out body reacts when food is consumed? With the parasympathetic nervous system suppressed (the part of the nervous system responsible for maintaining the body's homeostasis), both digestion and absorption are compromised. This is why indigestion, ulcers and irritable bowel syndrome are more common during stressful times.

This state of flux in which testosterone and cortisol vie for supremacy is known as the 'cortisol testosterone hormonal axis' and is linked to all sorts of changes in our behaviour and outlook. It's been shown, for example, that cortisol blocks some of the beneficial effects of testosterone. At the University of Texas [4], psychologists measured the hormone levels of saliva samples provided by 57 male subjects. The men were asked to take part in a one-on-one competition and were given the opportunity to compete again after winning or losing. Among those who lost, 100 per cent of the subjects with high testosterone and low cortisol requested a rematch, in an attempt to recapture their lost status. However, all of the participants with high testosterone and high cortisol levels who won declined to compete again. And the subjects who declined a rematch experienced a significant drop in testosterone after their initial defeat.

Another study at Harvard University [5] found that managers with greater leadership responsibility had higher levels of testosterone, associated with leadership qualities like aggressiveness and risk-taking, and low levels of cortisol. However, the authors concluded that stress can inhibit the leadership qualities associated with high levels of testosterone. Of course, stress also triggers behavioural changes that compound the hormonal slide – 46 per cent of people eat unhealthily or too much when they are stressed, 29 per cent start drinking or up their alcohol intake and 16 per cent take up smoking for the first time or increase the number of cigarettes smoked daily [3].

For all of these reasons, reducing stress levels in our lives is crucial for our wellbeing. And the pay-off could be improvements in low testosterone symptoms like rock-bottom libido, low energy and depression.

Did you know?

City traders who have high morning testosterone levels make more than average profits for the rest of that day, according to a study at the University of Cambridge [6]. It was suggested this is because of testosterone's ability to increase confidence and appetite for risk.

And Breathe ...

How we breathe is so instinctive that we do it without stopping to think. And yet it has a bearing on our stress levels, our hormones and our health. Take a deep breath and read on . . .

We spend so much time rushing around, looking at our smartphones and generally being distracted that we pay little attention to the most important thing we do as human beings: breathe. Scientists are only just beginning to look at how breathing affects our health, but they are already certain that poor habits have an impact on stress chemicals and, in turn, hormone levels. To find out more, researchers at the Medical University of South Carolina divided 20 healthy adults into two groups. One group was asked to perform two sets of simple 10-minute breathing exercises, while the other group was told to read a book or magazine of their choice for 20 minutes. Researchers took saliva swabs at various intervals during the exercise and their results showed [7] that the breathing exercise group had significantly lower levels of three cytokines that are associated with inflammation and stress.

Mindful or coherent breathing is a simple and great way to reduce stress in your life. Practise this approach for several minutes a day, gradually building up the time:

→ **Sit upright or lie down.**
→ **Place your hands on your stomach.**
→ **Slowly breathe in, expanding your belly, to the count of five.**
→ **Pause.**
→ **Slowly breathe out to the count of six.**

Work your way up to doing this breathing exercise for 10 to 15 minutes a day.

The meditation connection

Focusing on the present, as you do when you meditate, rather than letting the mind drift may help to lower levels of the stress hormone cortisol, which indirectly aids your testosterone and growth hormone levels. This, in turn, makes muscle building easier, and allows for a shorter recovery time after exercise. What's not to like about that proposal?

There's plenty of science to prove it works. When researchers from Johns Hopkins University sifted through nearly 19,000 meditation studies, they found 47 trials that met their criteria for well-designed studies and, from these, concluded [8] that mindful meditation can help ease psychological stresses like anxiety, depression and pain.

Many studies focus on the hormonal effects of the practice. In the Shamantha Project, a long-term, control-group study of the effects of meditation training on mind and body that was conducted at the University of California, researchers found [9] a correlation between a high score for mindfulness and a low score in cortisol both before and after a meditation retreat. Individuals whose mindfulness score increased after the retreat showed a decrease in cortisol. A study at Rutgers University [10] revealed that meditators have, on average, nearly a 50 per cent reduction in cortisol levels compared to non-meditators. Even more impressively, results can be seen within a couple of weeks. There's also increased activity of telomerase, an enzyme important for the long-term health of body cells.

Meditation works best in combination with exercise, especially when it comes to boosting mood. Men and women who completed an eight-week program combining exercise and meditation reported fewer depressive symptoms and said they did not spend as much time worrying about negative situations taking place in their lives as they did before the study began [10]. Incorporating meditation after a workout is a really great idea - not only will it help to reduce any exercise-induced cortisol, but it will allow for testosterone and post-workout protein synthesis to be elevated.

How to meditate

One of the best ways to lower your stress levels is to meditate daily. This is not some form of quackery, but has proven benefits. Mindful meditation can be as simple as sitting comfortably, focusing on your breathing, and then bringing your mind's attention to the present without drifting into concerns about the past or future.

Sit down: The trick to meditating on a chair is to ensure that your buttocks are somewhat higher than your knees. This tilts your pelvis forward and will help to keep your back nice and straight.

Ensure that your feet are flat on the ground, and your knees bent at 90 degrees.

Relax your hands: You can either have your hands on your thighs or folded in your lap. Relax your shoulders and, if at all possible, sit on the edge of the chair with your head aligned over your spine. If your spine needs additional support, feel free to put a cushion behind your back.

Use an app: When starting out, it can be beneficial to follow a guided audio. There are several free apps with progressive meditation audios available, and you may find you are able to settle into the practice quickly.

Count your breath: It is recommended that you start with 'counting the breath' meditation once or twice a day for two weeks, before moving on to 'following the breath' for two weeks, ending with 'practice of presence'.

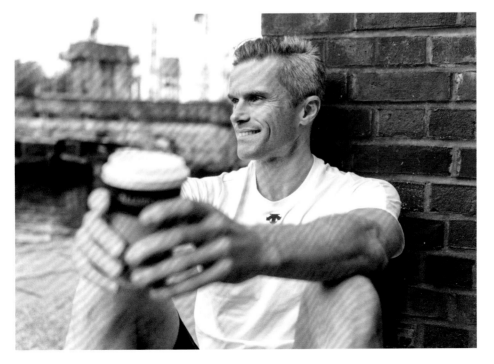

We all need to find a moment in the day to just take some time out, escape the treadmill of life, and let the mind wander and the body breathe.

Boost your Sex Drive

A sagging libido is often the first sign that a man's hormone levels are in decline. It can have a devastating effect on self-esteem and relationships. So, don't settle for a sex drive below par

Your sex drive (and your performance in the bedroom) can plummet as hormone levels decline. Who wouldn't want to prevent that? One of the welcome side-effects of the exercise and eating programme in this book is that it will almost certainly help to boost a flagging libido. Men who have tried the training programme have told me how, somewhat unexpectedly, their sex lives have improved as they have become fitter and stronger. But knowing there is research to support it, I am never surprised at their reports of much improved bedroom activity. Let's look at why this happens.

As we know, testosterone is a key male sex hormone involved in maintaining sex drive, erectile function and sperm production. It doesn't work alone, but in triggering the biological urges that sooner or later result in sex, it is essential for the survival of our species. However, following a peak in our late teens, testosterone levels begin their gradual decline after the age of 30. During our 40s and 50s, and more so by 60, many men notice that their sex drive is not what it was when they were more youthful. It may take longer to reach an erection, to achieve an orgasm and experience ejaculation. Erectile dysfunction becomes more common. No longer having the desire or the inclination for sex means that intimate relationships and self-confidence suffer as a consequence.

Previously, men have accepted this as an inevitable side-effect of ageing, something that can't be avoided unless you resort to chemical medication. But a growing number of scientists believe that our lifestyles, diet and fitness play much more of a crucial role in maintaining a healthy libido than was once thought. Certainly, there are reams of scientific evidence suggesting that re-booting your testosterone levels can help to reignite your sex life.

Proof that testosterone boosts your libido

In one of the first papers [11] from the Testosterone Trials (TTrials), a series of seven studies examining the effect of testosterone therapy in men, Yale University researchers collaborated with scientists at 12 other institutions to carry out trials that tested the efficacy of testosterone gel for, among other things, sexual function and vitality. They found that men who received testosterone therapy for one year, versus those on placebo, saw significant improvements in their sexual activity, sexual desire and erectile function.

Another placebo-controlled, double blind trial at Baylor College of Medicine, USA [12], examined the effect of testosterone therapy on sexual function in a group of 470 men aged 65 or older. All of the men had a heterosexual partner and, at the start of the study, all had been diagnosed with low testosterone levels. For this year-long test, the men were given a testosterone gel or a placebo applied to the skin and were asked to answer questionnaires about their sex lives every three months. Results clearly showed that the testosterone therapy boosted sex drive and in 10 of the 12 sexual activity measurements assessed, including frequency of intercourse, masturbation and night time erections. Men who didn't get their testosterone charged experienced no such changes.

Why health, fitness and lifestyle matter

These studies prove that testosterone can reverse a flagging sex drive. But I am certainly not advocating therapy via medication, patches or gels. Decades ago, researchers discovered that, for men, exercise is key to a better sex life. Men who completed fairly intense exercise three to five days a week were shown to develop 'significantly greater sexual enhancements' [13] which included a higher percentage of satisfying orgasms. What scientists now know is that our health and fitness play a much greater role in preserving men's libido as they age than was once thought. They have nailed down precisely what type of exercise best boosts declining hormones – and it is those included within this book. Whereas hefty endurance training (marathons and long-distance cycling), high levels of stress and over-training for your age can cause testosterone to plummet to worrying levels, adversely affecting your sex drive, a combination of resistance and high intensity training will go a long way towards boosting them. Combined with the testosterone-boosting diet I advocate, your sex drive will only be heading in one direction.

Why relationships matter

In the longer term, you may find that you are on a roll. Gary Wittert, Professor of Medicine at the University of Adelaide, Australia, and his team analysed the testosterone levels in more than 1,500 male recruits who ranged in age from 35 to 80 years, with an average age of 54 [13]. The men were asked to two clinic visits five years apart to have their testosterone levels measured via a blood test. What was observed over the five-year study was that unmarried men (or those not in a relationship) had greater testosterone reductions than married men. Previous research had also shown that men in relationships tend to be healthier and happier than single men, but also that sexual activity itself

increased testosterone. In other words, the more sex you have with a partner, the greater the boost to your testosterone. A win-win situation if ever there was one.

Speed Read

→ Our hectic lifestyles are responsible for rising stress levels and consequent hormonal disruption.

→ The stress hormone, cortisol, works against testosterone, adversely changing our mental and physical behaviour.

→ Stress can cause hormonal changes that trigger low testosterone symptoms, such as flagging energy, low libido and susceptibility to illness.

→ Breathing mindfully is a great way to combat stress.

→ Daily meditation can lower levels of cortisol and works in tandem with exercise to create a positive hormonal equilibrium.

→ Your sex drive improves as hormonal levels are restored.

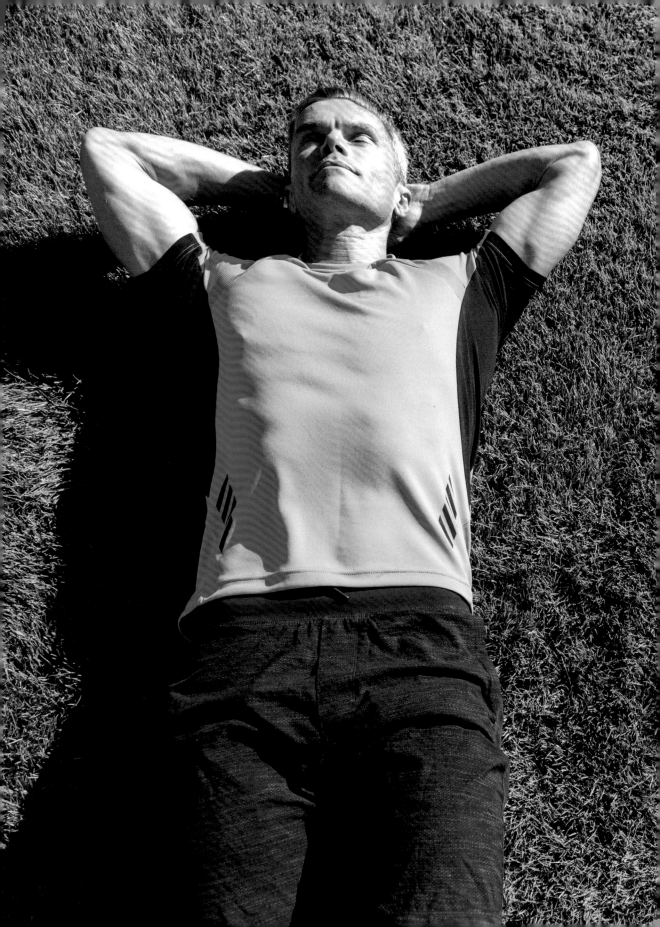

Sleep and Recovery

For all the effort you will be making in the gym over the next two months, there is an essential aspect of my programme that involves you doing very little at all. Recovery is all-important for the building of muscles and the production of hormones that lead to a younger-looking, fitter and stronger body. As you will see in this chapter, recovery and sleep are vital for health. Without them, you simply won't progress in the way that is possible.

The Power of Sleep

At no time of day or night is our hormone production more active than when we are asleep. Fail to get enough shut-eye – as many of us do – and we are on a slippery slope. Don't underestimate sleep's power

Giving ourselves enough sleep of the right quality is truly an integral part of good health. It affects your metabolism, blood pressure, energy, ability to concentrate, immune system, mood, and just about every other aspect of your health – recovery and hormone production included.

While we are asleep our bodies are busily running a number of different processes that are vital to ensure we bounce back the next day. Sleep research has demonstrated that the brain is as active as ever during sleep: information is processed, memories are created and stored; toxins are cleaned out of brain tissue; and, of course, the parts of the brain responsible for breathing and other necessary functions never take a break. Hormones and extra protein molecules are released during sleep which work to strengthen your immune system and help your body repair itself from a multitude of ills, including stress, pollutants and infection. Your body also processes toxins and provides energy to organs while you sleep. And it is at night that the hormones that affect and control your appetite are regulated.

When you consider that sleep is something we spend nearly a third of our lives doing, we really should be very good at it. Yet we are getting less sleep than ever. Research by the Royal Society for Public Health in 2016 found that we typically sleep for 6.8 hours a night, far less than the golden goal of 8 hours a night purported to be essential for health. And this lack of shut-eye is undoubtedly affecting our health. A lack of sleep raises your body's levels of the hunger hormone leptin meaning you will crave sugary, carb-based foods, which are often processed. Poor sleep quality also affects productivity, job satisfaction and career progression. We are more negative and willing to take risks when we are tired. As our energy levels drop, so too does our aptitude and inclination for exercise. A lesser known impact of chronic sleep deprivation is that it affects the very male hormones we are trying to boost with my 8-week plan. Let's look at how and why this happens.

The hormone effect

There are various phases of sleep, the most physically restorative being non-REM (rapid eye movement) deep sleep, when your blood pressure drops and your breathing becomes deeper and slower. During this phase, your brain is resting with very little activity and with reduced need for blood supply. This means that more blood is available for your muscles and tissues and it's at this point that extra amounts of oxygen and nutrients offering potential for healing and growth are delivered. Huge amounts of regeneration take place within your cells during this phase of sleep, but something else occurs to bring further benefit. At night, your pituitary gland, a kidney-bean-sized gland in the brain, releases a shot of HGH which flows into your bloodstream and stimulates further tissue growth and muscle repair.

It stands to reason that, if all this happens when you are in the land of nod, then a lack of sleep or changes in your usual sleep quality cause the

Matt Says:

The hormones controlling our appetite are regulated at night, while we sleep

opposite to happen – namely, a sharp decline in HGH secretion. Getting too little sleep drastically reduced young men's testosterone levels in one study: at the University of Chicago [1], sleep researchers found that men who slept less than five hours a night for one week in a laboratory had significantly lower levels of testosterone than when they had a full night's sleep. And the effects of sleep loss on testosterone levels were apparent after just one week of short sleep. Five hours of sleep decreased their testosterone levels by 10 to 15 per cent. The young men had the lowest testosterone levels in the afternoons on their sleep-restricted days between 2pm and 10pm. Unsurprisingly, the men also reported their mood and energy dropped throughout the study, as too did their sense of well-being as their blood testosterone levels plummeted.

Performance-limiting

Lots of research has been conducted at Stanford University's sleep disorders clinic [2] where, for one study, the sleep/wake patterns of five athletes were tracked over three weeks during which time they were asked to perform a series of athletic tests that included sprinting, tennis serves and other drills. On average, the athletes were getting between six to eight hours' sleep a night, not much considering their training levels. When the same subjects were asked to extend their sleeping hours to ten per night, their performance in the drills improved significantly and they were able to run faster, hit tennis balls more accurately and exhibit greater arm strength. This suggests that people who are more active may benefit from nine to 10 hours' sleep, more than the average person gets per night in

the UK. A University of California study [3] showed that injury rates in young athletes increased during games that followed a night of fewer than six hours' sleep. A different study [4] suggested that sleep hours were a stronger predictor of injuries in athletes than hours of practice and training.

Did you know?

Eat Greek yoghurt before bed. During the seven to 10 hours you are asleep, the body is primed for recovery, so take advantage of boosting training adaptations by eating Greek yoghurt 30 minutes before hitting the sack. The protein in yoghurt and other milk products is almost entirely casein, which digests slowly in the body and is ideal for rebuilding muscle following any intense training training session, but particularly a gym workout using weights. In 2012, a study by Professor Luc van Loon from Maastricht University demonstrated that consuming casein after a strength workout and half an hour before going to bed stimulated muscle protein synthesis overnight much better than a placebo.

Sleep Stages

Not all sleep is the same and we drift in and out of sleep stages that are of different duration and quality. Tracking your sleep patterns can help you to understand more

Scientists have identified five stages of sleep and the amount of time we spend in each stage is vital to get fully restorative sleep. Age, gender, health and lifestyle all play a major part in how long we spend in each stage of sleep. Finding the best ways of increasing our stage 3 and 4 sleep is the answer to real quality sleep and all the benefits that come with it.

Stage 1: The stage between awake and asleep, also includes very light sleep.

Stage 2: Fully asleep, breathing and heart rate steady, body temperature drops slightly.

Stage 3 and 4: Deep and restorative sleep, muscles relaxed, energy restored, hormones released.

REM (Rapid Eye Movement): Dream stage, usually occurs about 90 minutes after falling asleep and then again a few more times, with each REM stage lasting a little longer than the one before it.

Should you track your sleep?

Understanding how we sleep and what habits, choices, foods and environments help us get better sleep is essential. Regularly collating a sleep diary is a great way of understanding how to make the most of this essential part of the day. Each morning recording the quality of sleep that you feel you have had and how recovered you feel is the start of the process to understanding the effectiveness of your sleep. Alternatively, you could use a sleep tracker or app.

Technology has provided some wonderful innovations that can aid your fitness and health. I am a big fan of devices that tally the amount of sleep you have totted up each night. I find that keeping tabs on my sleep patterns is a very clear indicator of how rested or how stressed I am. As digital health devices become more high-tech, featuring sensitive heart-rate monitors that use night-time heart-rate data to estimate light, deep and REM sleep, or claim to capture variables such as movement, humidity, breathing patterns and temperature information to assess your sleep, accuracy has improved, but they are far from infallible.

You need to be careful that sleep tracking is used as a guide to improve health and that it doesn't become an obsession in itself. Researchers at Rush University and the Feinberg School of medicine at Northwestern University [5] have dubbed a growing obsession for sleep measurement 'orthosomnia' and their findings suggest that sleep trackers can do more harm than good, interfering with your hours of restful sleep rather than improving them.

Matt Says:

Keeping track of my sleep gives me a clear indicator of how stressed I am feeling

Sleep and Working Out

When you exercise can influence your sleep quantity and quality. And while activity can help you to get to sleep more easily, more of it is not always better

If you do have trouble sleeping, the good news is that your insomnia may improve once you embark on this 8-week plan. Countless studies have shown that a single bout of moderate-intensity aerobic exercise (even walking) can reduce the time it takes for those with chronic insomnia to fall asleep and increase the length of time spent asleep. Regular exercise helps to normalise our body clock (circadian rhythm) and therefore makes it more likely that your eyes will be closing by the time your head hits the pillow. People who are active before bed are generally more efficient sleepers, according to research published; they also fell asleep faster, slept deeper, and woke up less during the night.

If you have not been doing any exercise recently, scheduling your workouts for the afternoon or early evening may help initially. However, be careful not to exercise too vigorously, too close to bedtime. Intense exercise can lead to the elevation of certain hormones (such as cortisol) that may prevent you drifting off to sleep. It is best to do your hardest workouts earlier in the day, making sure you allow for at least three to four hours before you go to bed.

Beware overtraining

Let's make a clear distinction between effort and overdoing it. I am asking you to work hard in the eight weeks you will be following my plan, but that doesn't mean I haven't factored in recovery; a failure to do that would be counterproductive. Putting in maximum effort every day will lead you down a fast route to overtraining and the effects can be catastrophic, not least for your sleep patterns. While an optimum amount of exercise may help improve your sleep, too much will likely disrupt it.

There are many studies that prove you can't go hard at exercise all the time. In one [6], Jinger Gottschall, Assistant Professor of Kinesiology at Penn State University, USA, recruited 35 healthy adults who typically worked out for more than eight hours a week and asked them to wear a heart rate monitor while carrying out their usual exercise routine for three weeks. They were also asked to keep tabs on their diet and mood.

Results showed a direct correlation between time spent training at a high intensity of 90 per cent maximum heart rate and what scientists call 'overreaching', symptoms of which included disrupted sleep, more illness and injury, and a plateau or drop in fitness.

There is simply no direct correlation between continued maximum effort and weight lost or definition gained. If you are training intensely every day, you could find you hit a plateau where your fitness doesn't improve.

Fitter = Faster Recovery

Exercise scientists place recovery high on the agenda for athletes and have invested much time and effort in finding the best ways to do it. Their findings apply to all of us

There's good news, however: following my 8-week programme will speed up the relative ease with which you bounce back for your next session. Because even with age, the fitter you are the faster you will recover from a hard workout. This was demonstrated in a study at the University of Central Florida, USA, [7], that compared the recovery responses of nine men with an average age of 22 to ten men with an average age of 47. All participants, young and old, were fit and had been performing resistance workouts for at least six months prior to taking part. To find out how different their powers of recovery were, researchers got all of the men to perform a 'high-volume isokinetic resistance exercise' workout – 8 sets of 10 repetitions using machines where they straightened and then flexed the knee against a resistance – while blood samples were taken to analyse the muscle damage and inflammation that occurred.

You might have expected the youngsters to have recovered their powers of strength more readily, but results displayed no differences between the two groups. Granted, the younger subjects were stronger to begin with, but the relative loss and recovery of strength was the same in all men, whatever their age. Interestingly, they also displayed the same markers of stress and inflammation and reported similar effects of pain and soreness.

OK, so it's proven: as you get fitter, you'll recover faster. But how can you ensure that you recover most effectively? For starters, follow my six steps to better sleep hygiene:

1_Get up at the same time
Getting up at the same time each day can help to regulate sleep patterns. A study published in the journal *Scientific Reports* found that students [8]

who did not go to bed or wake up at consistent times every day were more likely to have lower grades. Hitting the snooze button for a weekend lie-in is not the answer. A one-hour lie-in at weekends was enough to cause 'social jet lag', a phemonenon caused by a discrepancy between your body's internal clock and your sleep schedule, that is linked to mood swings and fatigue.

2_Try cryotherapy
You've probably seen images of top athletes apparently aiding their recovery process by jumping into a tub of icy water. This is a form of 'cryotherapy', a medical practice that involves exposure to very cold temperatures. Studies have shown that submerging yourself in an ice bath reduces perceptions of soreness and speeds up the recovery of muscle function, although not everyone agrees. Researchers at Liverpool John Moores University, UK, [9] have concluded that ice baths are no better than an 'active recovery' (walking about a bit and doing some stretching) in terms of fighting post-workout inflammation.

What we do know is that cryotherapy can trigger the activity of creatine kinase, an important enzyme in muscle tissue that has a proven anti-ageing effect and is an indicator of muscle damage. Researchers [10] measured muscle pain, tiredness and quadriceps strength, and collected blood samples from a group of trained athletes to test their muscle damage. Specifically, the scientists measured levels of creatine kinase (CK), which leaks from damaged muscle into the blood stream, following two hard workouts, one followed by a cryotherapy session. Ratings of muscle pain and tiredness were reduced after the first cryotherapy session.

3_Don't take your smartphone to bed

Your smartphone, laptop, tablet and television are all best avoided for at least 45 minutes before you go to bed. They all emit short wavelength, blue light that suppresses melatonin and fools the brain into thinking it is daytime. Using them also means you are doing something that is keeping the brain alert, not helpful when trying to drift off to sleep.

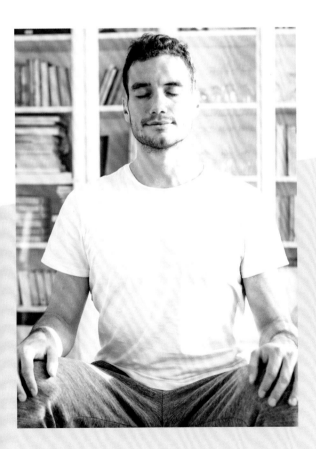

4_Make sure your room is quiet and dark

A bedroom that is peaceful and dark is one in which you are much more likely to fall asleep. To achieve such an environment, try using earplugs to block out noise and heavy curtains to minimise light.

5_Keep your room at the right temperature

If you feel too hot or too cold, you are more likely to wake up during the night. Your body temperature peaks in the evening and then drops to its lowest levels when you're asleep, meaning any draught could wake you up. The optimum temperature for sleeping is 16-18°C, while temperatures over 24°C are likely to cause restlessness. A cold room of about 12°C is probably too cool and you'll be fidgeting to keep warm rather than dropping off into a restful slumber. Remember to make tweaks to your environment in summer or winter, such as leaving a window open if it's warm, or changing the tog of your duvet, to achieve the right sleeping temperature.

6_Try Magnesium Salt Baths

Having a warm, not hot, bath with magnesium flakes has been proven to relax the muscles and in turn relax the whole body. This then allows us to fall asleep quicker and prevents tension in the body disturbing our sleep during the night.

→ 7 Ways to Eat your Way to Sleep

If you are still having trouble dropping off at night, there are also nutritional steps you can take to improve your sleep duration. Try some of the following to see if you can get to sleep more easily

1_Avoid caffeine before bed

Since its stimulating effects can last for several hours, even one caffeinated drink can make it hard to nod off or cause you to wake up in the middle of the night. Researchers from the Sleep Disorders & Research Centre at the Henry Ford Hospital in Detroit, USA, [11] gave a group of volunteers a dose of caffeine at their usual bedtime or three and six hours beforehand. Their results, reported in the *Journal of Clinical Sleep Medicine*, concluded that caffeine consumed within six hours of going to bed has disruptive effects on sleep.

2_Don't use alcohol as a sleep cure

Alcohol lulls people into a false sense of sleep security. You may fall asleep more quickly after a glass or two of wine, but it's likely that you will wake up in the middle of the night when the effects wear off. Alcohol disrupts your entire sleep cycle so that your heart rate is elevated and you spend more time awake. You are also likely to feel parched and wake up to get a drink.

3_Take 5-HTP

The compound 5-hydroxytryptophan (or 5-HTP) is made naturally in the body and created as a by-product of the amino acid L-tryptophan. Available as a supplement, 5-HTP helps the body to produce serotonin, a neurotransmitter that helps to regulate our sleep-wake cycles. Research suggests that 5-HTP may help reduce the time it takes to fall asleep and increase the amount of time you spend asleep [12].

4_Increase your GABA levels

People with chronic insomnia have been shown to have 30 per cent lower levels of GABA, a neurotransmitter used to dampen nerve activity in the brain and promote deep relaxation, than good sleepers. Some people find a supplement of GABA helpful, but you can also consume a diet rich in foods that contain glutamate, a substance that helps to optimise your GABA levels. Glutamate-high foods include eggs and poultry, cheese, sea vegetables, ripe tomatoes and mushrooms. Fermented foods, vegetables and kefir are rich in certain beneficial bacteria that also have a marked impact on your GABA levels.

Matt Says:

Sleep is vital to our processes of recovery, repair and re-energising. Skimp and your body will suffer

5_Drink green tea during the day

Green tea contains L-theanine, an amino acid that crosses your blood-brain barrier and is said to have psychoactive properties. It is known to increase levels of serotonin, dopamine and alpha brainwave activity as well as reduce mental and physical stress, and has been shown to aid sleep [13]. However, remember that green tea does contain caffeine and if you are susceptible to its effects, you should avoid it just before bedtime

6_Eat oily fish

There are many health reasons to eat oily fish, such as salmon and tuna, and better sleep can be added to that list. Sleep problems in children have been linked to behavioural and cognitive issues, problems also associated with deficiencies of the omega 3 fatty acids found in oily fish. For a study at the University of Oxford, researchers recruited 362 children, some of whom had clinical sleep problems, who were given either a 600 mg supplement of omega 3 or a placebo. Results showed that those taking the fish oils gained an extra hour's sleep and had seven fewer waking episodes each night.

7_Eat fruit

Plenty of researchers have linked impaired sleep with low antioxidant levels. Fruit is a great way to boost your intake of antioxidants, and some appear to be more beneficial than others. A month-long study of 24 volunteers with sleep problems [14] revealed that volunteers slept 13 per cent longer if they ate two kiwi fruits an hour before bed each night. Although the precise reasons why kiwi fruit acts as a sedative aren't known, it could be down to the high antioxidant levels in the fruit. Kiwis are also high in serotonin, a hormone that's critical to sleep, and which can help to increase levels of the so-called 'sleep hormone', melatonin, in the body. Pineapples, oranges and bananas have also been linked to improved sleep for similar reasons.

Why Heart Rate Matters

Keeping tabs on your heart rate is a reliable way
to determine how hard (or not) you are working
and how well (or not) you are recovering

Your resting heart rate (the number of beats per minute your heart makes when lying down at rest) is a measure of how efficiently your heart works. A lower resting heart rate implies more efficient heart function and better cardiovascular fitness. So, a top athlete might have a resting heart rate close to just 40 beats per minute whereas a 'normal' resting heart rate for other adults can range from 60 to 100 beats per minute. As you get fitter, your heart gets stronger and your heart can pump more blood with one beat. In 'other words, your 'stroke volume' improves.

Your resting heart rate is easy to measure: place your index and middle finger on your wrist just below the thumb, or along either side of your neck, so you can feel your pulse, and, using a watch, count the number of beats for 30 seconds, double it to get your beats per minute.

Maximum heart rate

Your maximum heart rate – the most beats per minute that you can reach through physical effort – is largely genetically predetermined and won't change dramatically over time. Though your heart will become stronger and more efficient as you get fitter, pumping out more blood per beat and allowing you to do more at the same heart rate, the closer you are to your max heart rate during exercise, the less time you will be able to keep up that level of effort.

There are basic formulas for working out your maximum heart rate – among the most common is 220 minus your age – but they are inaccurate and only a very rudimentary guide.

Heart rate variability

A healthy heart beat contains healthy irregularities. Even if your resting heart rate is, say, 60 beats per minute, it doesn't mean that your heart beats once every second – or at exact one-second intervals like a digital clock. For all of us, there is some degree of variation among the intervals between our heartbeats and this might vary from 0.85 seconds between two succeeding beats to 1.35 seconds between some others. Your heart rate variability (HRV) is controlled by the autonomic nervous system (ANS) and it indicates quite how much variation, measured in milliseconds (ms), there is in your heartbeats within a specific time frame.

Generally, a low HRV (or less variability in the heart beats) suggests your body is under some sort of stress from exercise, psychological events, or other internal or external stressors. Higher HRV (or greater variability between heart beats) tends to indicate your body has a strong ability to tolerate stress or recovers well from physical stress. It's worth bearing in mind that your HRV is unique and it's unwise to start comparing levels with others. It is a measure that is affected by age, hormones and overall body functions, as well as what you eat and how you exercise, and women typically have an HRV higher than men.

Researchers and physiologists have been tracking and utilising HRV for decades because it's a useful indicator of several health-related issues. They have found it matters because a low HRV has been linked with a higher risk of heart disease [15] and to a lower risk of death [16, 17] in older people. I find HRV is a really good indicator of the state of my clients' health and fitness, recovery and rested state. It can tell you many things:

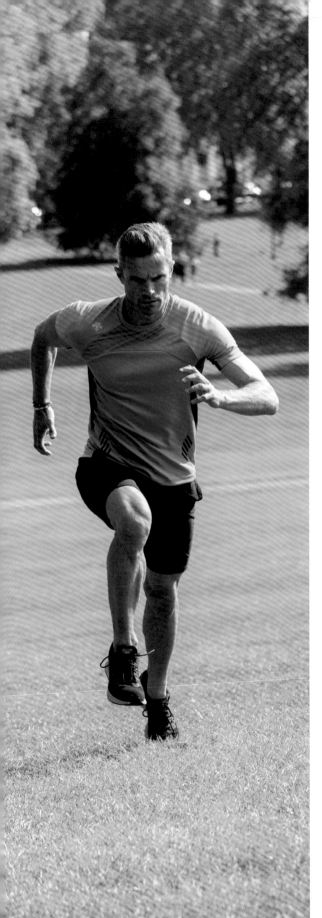

→ Stress and lack of sleep can cause your HRV to drop, indicating that you might need to take some time out for recovery.

→ During and just after intensive training, your HRV can drop sharply [18, 19, 20]. If you recover well, it will bounce back to normal, suggesting you are fit enough to cope with the training load. If your HRV doesn't return to normal quickly, you may have been overreaching or are overtraining.

→ Your HRV can drop just before you fall sick and often before you have any symptoms. It is a clear sign that you are run down.

→ Your HRV will plummet if you smoke or if you drink more than usual.

→ Dehydration can cause your HRV to drop temporarily (although it will return to normal once you are hydrated).

The easiest and cheapest way to check your HRV is to buy a heart rate chest-strap monitor and to download an app, such as Elite HRV, to analyse the data. I advise checking your HRV in the mornings after you wake up a few times a week, and then tracking for changes as you progress through the 8-week plan.

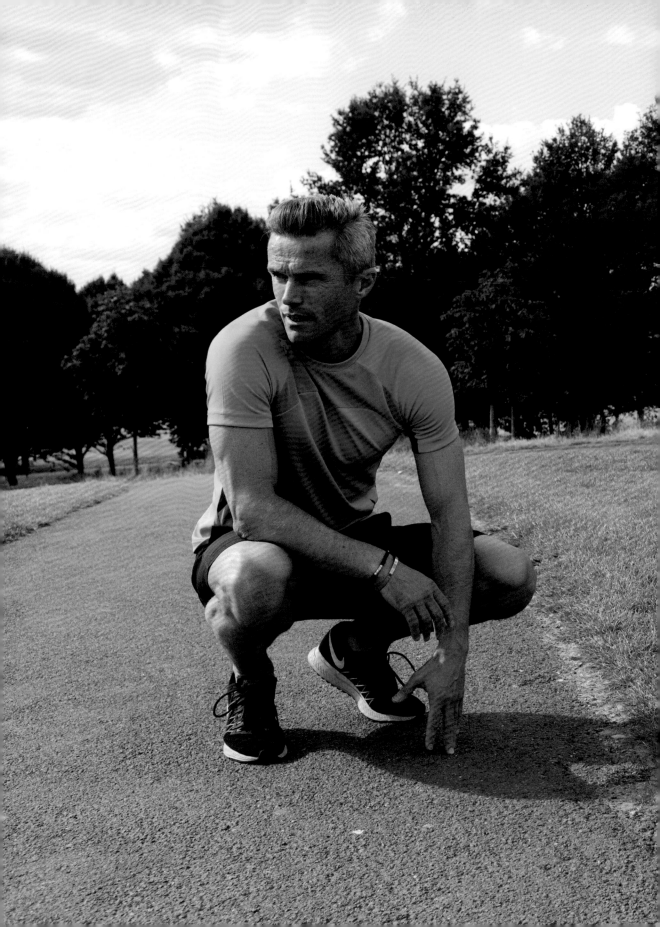

Chapter Eight

Motivation and Planning

One of the hardest things about getting fitter is getting started. This is a universal truth and it is also a factor that sees many people hang up the towel before they have even gotten underway with a new programme. Let's make no bones about it, this programme is no walkover. It will require dedication, sweat and perseverance, but you will be rewarded for your efforts and your patience.

Setting and Maintaining Goals

Your body can only respond to change if your mind is prepared for it. And motivation is key to that process. Here I outline ways to get yourself mentally ready for the task ahead

When I work with my clients, I like to sit down and talk to them about their goals. What is really driving them to get fitter and stronger? What was the trigger that made them want to change their lives? And where do they see themselves a month, a year and a decade from now? Sticking to this 8-week programme will be so much easier if you have a clear idea of where you want it to take you. And goal-setting is something that I encourage you to do before you get started, too.

Sit down with a notepad and jot down what it is you'd like to achieve – in the long and the short term – from this programme. For some of you this will take moments. You will know instantly that you want to lose the pounds around your middle or to become healthier so that you can take part in a football match with your kids. But for others it might be a case of creating a goal. 'If I get rid of these moobs, I will…' or 'I want to complete every exercise I am set', for example.

Remember that goals are supposed to be personal. It's no point sharing someone else's goal or you will eventually lack the motivation to achieve it. And no goal is too small. If all you want to achieve by the end of this is to feel happier about yourself, then that is admirable in itself. Give yourself rewards too: when you meet a mini-milestone, congratulate yourself with a new pair of trainers or a nice meal.

Along the way, there are bound to be times when your motivation dips. Even the most diligent and aspirational exercisers periodically hit these low points when they begin to question what and why they are doing something. Work through it because I promise you it will be worth it.

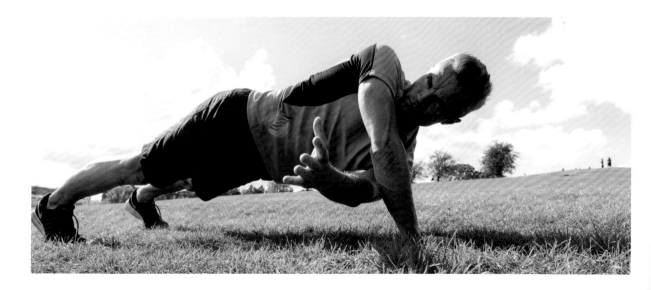

→ How to Measure your Progress

One of the best ways to motivate yourself is to keep tabs on how far you have come since you started. I advise all of my clients to do this

Measuring change and being motivated by the ongoing improvements you can see is a really important part of the programme. Bear in mind that this programme has multiple goal outcomes – you want to look and feel younger, fitter and stronger – so there is no single measurement that will provide an accurate marker for your progress. Think about it: we are looking to make you physically stronger, aiming to reduce fat storage on the body and make you leaner, make you posturally stronger and more mobile, and aiming to help your body deal with stress and the increased ageing effect on the body. There are a lot of factors for improvement and you may find that some occur more quickly than others. Progress is always individual, but here are some pointers as to how you can check things are heading in the right direction:

Strength gains

This one is fairly simple to evaluate. Writing down the amount of weight that you can move tells you exactly how much stronger you are getting. Chart your strength developments and perhaps create a line graph to show the strength uplift on each exercise. This measured strength improvement is what will keep you strong for a long healthy life and help maintain strong bones and joints.

Cosmetic gains

Charting your cosmetic changes can be done in a number of ways. At the simplest level, you can feel the difference on your body in the fit of your clothes. Be aware of what is becoming tighter and what feels like it is fitting more loosely. On the programme I would expect you to feel that you are losing fat from your mid-section, but gaining muscle across your back and chest. I would certainly expect your legs to feel stronger and the muscles around your bottom to be bigger. You can also measure change more precisely: using a measuring tape, take measurements across your chest, middle of your upper arm, around your waist just below your belly button and middle of your thigh. Keep taking these measurements every couple of weeks and chart the changes. Taking pictures of yourself in the mirror and see what change is happening is another option. The only measure I wouldn't take is weight as this will not give you a true indication of progression as you gain muscle and strength.

Mobility gains

You be able to feel mobility developing as you progress through this programme. Every time you do the Couch Stretch (page 99) or the 90/90 Hip Stretch (page 98) you should feel how much better you can perform it and how much more movement you have.

→ Perils of Socialising

A pitfall of many a good intention is a night out with friends or colleagues. Having fun is an essential part of life/work balance and an important form of stress relief. Just ensure you don't socialise to excess

What happens when you want a night out? Will your good intentions come crashing down and your hopes of a younger, fitter and stronger body be dashed? Not necessarily.

Meeting with friends, family and work colleagues to socialise is an important part of life and one of the factors that keeps us young, helps prime our mental focus and helps us de-stress. However, we need to control the amount of socialising we do, especially when it involves the food and alcohol that can go hand in hand with social events. While you are on the programme, I suggest you keep nights, and lunches, out to a minimum. You have committed to this programme and need to be focused if you are to fully reap the benefits that come from it. Don't be concerned that you will fall out of the loop or that friends and colleagues will see you differently. In my experience of working with clients who were very concerned about cutting down on social engagements, the opposite was true – they found that people were impressed that they were following a controlled 8-week programme and respected the changes they were trying to make. And the same will almost certainly be true for you. But if you do go out, stick to your guns and don't veer away from your diet plan. All too often I hear clients tell me how they felt under pressure to drink alcohol when they went out, but actually, you will be amazed how many people are happy to go out to get some healthier food and drink less. Most of us just need someone else to lead us in the right direction. Also try socialising differently; rather than just going for drinks, go and play a sport and then have a drink. Work on balance in your life.

Motivational tips

Here are some of my top tips to help you stay focused and on track:

1_Remember your drivers: The starting point of achievement is your desire, the drivers that lead you to accept this challenge. Keep that in mind.

2_Prioritise yourself: Too many people fail to do this on a regular basis. You deserve nothing but the best and you have the power to be unstoppable. So, make sure you nourish yourself well, support yourself with sleep and recovery and empower yourself in the process. That way you can perform at your optimum level.

3_Master your body: There is only one person who has control of your body – and it is you. If you don't assume that control, then your capacity to maximise your health, energy and vitality will be compromised. Your body is amazing and you need it to be in top form so that you have the energy and passion to pursue everything in this life that you want to achieve.

4_Seek out small victories: A huge goal can seem unattainable – and at times overwhelming. It's good to have them, but make sure you keep focused by challenging yourself along the way with small goals. There's evidence that doing this builds new androgen receptors in the brain, areas responsible for reward and motivation. This increase in androgen receptors boosts the influence of testosterone, further increasing your confidence and desire to succeed. With a series of small victories, your confidence and motivation can be heightened for months on end.

5_Be consistent: Don't panic if you have to miss a workout – but don't make a habit of it. Consistency is key to fitness and strength gains for you to progress and achieve the body you desire.

6_Take 5: Self-reflection and introspection are important mental exercises that can help you to grow and I encourage all of my clients to spend five to 10 minutes daily just sitting back from their fast-paced lives to bring focus back where it belongs. We each have about 50,000 thoughts a day, over half of which are negative and almost 1,000 of which are repeats from the previous day. Take the time and effort to focus your mind in a positive direction and you will give yourself the opportunity to flourish.

7_Don't overlook recovery: Exercise is a stimulus for body improvement, but success comes from the way we recover. I can't stress enough how important it is to keep this in the forefront of your mind. Controlling and understanding the way my clients recover is incredibly important to their overall progression. Find ways and means to assist your own recovery through meditation, yoga, cryotherapy or just sitting down and reading a book.

8_Energise yourself through sleep: Remember that sleep is where we re-energise, recover and re-establish many of our body responses. Being able to consistently get enough sleep (seven-plus hours for most people) is essential both for these reasons but also to keep you motivated. When you are tired, you will lack the energy and drive to exercise or to follow your diet plan. Make sure you get enough.

9_Decide who you want to be: Instead of trying to answer the question 'Who am I?', try to answer the question 'Who am I becoming?' Decide who you need to be to be fitter, younger and stronger, and grow into that new persona.

10_Start the week determined, finish the week satisfied: This is a personal motto of mine that works to help me – and my clients – stay motivated. It can really help to break down your 8-week programme into manageable chunks of seven days of activity. And if you've had a bad weekend, get yourself straight back on track come Monday morning.

11_Manage your time well: Our time is precious and valuable – once you've wasted time you can't get it back. There are 168 hours in every week and you have an average 2,400 minutes to yourself each week. That is a monumental amount of time when you think about it. So much can be achieved in that time if you manage it well and let go of everything you don't want – or need – to do. Use your time well.

12_Don't be afraid of making mistakes: Always remember that no matter how many setbacks and how many mistakes you make along the way, you are still way ahead of anyone who isn't trying to improve.

Matt Says:

You are not a failure if you occasionally drift off course

Planning around Work and Family Life

Fitting in a new healthy living programme around your
job and kids is not always easy. But it can be done

Our lives are incredibly busy and by middle age
you can feel your attention and focus being pulled
in a hundred different directions. Of course, work
and family life are a priority and you should not let
your dedication to them slip, but how can you work
around the demands they place on you? Here are
my top three tips:

Plan ahead: Remember that the fitter you are, the
better it is for your work and your family. Therefore,
planning and looking after yourself becomes of
even greater importance. Instead of thinking of why
you can't fit in your workouts, think of ways you can.

Join in: Don't be one of those dads who simply
stands watching their children at football training,
chatting with a super-sized creamy coffee in their
hands, and never does any exercise themselves.
If your children are doing something active, plan to
do something active yourself. Take the time to pop
to the gym or do some running intervals. Use and
plan your time well and everyone's needs will be
catered for.

Don't feel guilty: Calculate the time needed for your
daily workouts and then decide when you can fit them
in to your day. This is not always easy and may take
some juggling, but there will be a convenient time
slot, even if it means rising extra early. By setting a
timetable like this in advance, you feel less guilty than
you would if you've dashed off to the gym when your
youngest needed taking to their piano lesson.

What if things go wrong?
Not everything goes to plan in life and you may find
that you slip behind with the programme or that you
fall off the wagon altogether. It's not the end of the
world, but how do you make amends?

Stay focused: One of the most important elements
to get right on the programme is to stay in tune with
your goals so that you have a focus every day. Take
time to make sure your week is planned so that you
have limited any potential faults within your week.

Take it day by day: I find that people can get
overwhelmed if they view a programme in its entirety
and if their ultimate goal seems a long way from
where they are right now. It's important to see each
day as a different part of the overall plan. That way,
if you miss one or two days, you don't consider
yourself a failure.

> **→ What if you get really hungry?**
> With the exception of the fasting days,
> you have a high-nutrient diet on this
> programme so you should not feel
> overwhelmingly hungry. If you do get
> feelings of hunger ask yourself if it really
> is hunger that you are experiencing.
> Sometimes we feel hungry because of
> boredom. Stress is another factor that
> makes us feel hungry; because of the
> 'fight or flight' reaction, we feel low in
> energy and confuse that with a need to
> eat. You may also mistake the sensation
> of thirst for hunger, so make sure that
> you stay hydrated right through the day.

Assess your progress: Checking your progress can really help to heighten your motivation levels (see page 86).

Have a plan B or C: Make sure that occasionally you have some plan Bs and even plan Cs for food and exercise. This will help to offset the guilt you feel when things do go wrong. If you are out for lunch and can't stick to your diet plan for the day, have a list of healthy options that you can eat in restaurants.

Learn from your experiences: If you fall off the plan, don't dwell on it, just get back on track and learn from what distracted you.

Remember to reflect: On the programme there will be days when you feel great and there will be days when you feel tired. Instead of just soldiering on, take a break and assess why you feel so exhausted. How did you sleep? How was your food intake yesterday? Was yesterday a hard training day? Is work stressful?

Take time to see if you can address any of these or if you are feeling tired because of tough training – which is perfectly normal. Think of ways you can redress the balance and get the recovery you need.

Can you have any treats?

Treats are a normal – I would even say an important – part of life. They are something we look forward to having and I would not be human if I didn't occasionally indulge (or allow my clients to do the same). However, the name speaks volumes: treats are a reward and they should be something that we plan towards and look forward to, not something that becomes the norm. If you have a treat – a glass of wine, a chocolate bar – every day, then by definition you are no longer treating yourself.

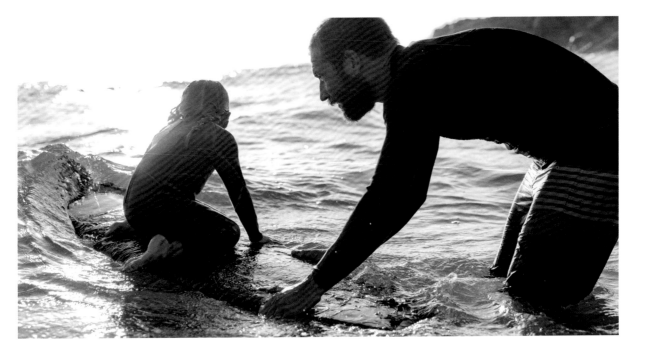

Safety

Don't skim past this page thinking it doesn't matter. Making sure you are familiar with the potential risks (there are few) of my exercise plan and that you are well versed in how to avoid them is crucial

---

Before you get started it's important to look at a few aspects of safety that will ensure you get the most out of your workouts and avoid injury.

 01 If you have any lingering injuries or medical conditions, do make sure you seek medical advice before embarking on my plan. Like any new programme it will require some drastic changes to your existing lifestyle and you need to know you are in a fit and healthy state to get going.

 02 Make sure you have a space that is big enough (and safe enough) to exercise in. For many of you, this will be a gym environment, but if you are lucky enough to have the equipment needed at home, make sure there are no slippy mats or rugs and that the room is well-ventilated and well lit.

 03 Make sure you familiarise yourself with each workout programme before attempting it. Read the exercise descriptions thoroughly, especially if you are trying new moves.

04 Give equipment the once over before you use it. Weights can become loose and machines can be poorly stacked. While this may be through no fault of your own, you may be the one who suffers the consequences.

 05 Wipe equipment down before using it. Sweat can make weights very slippery and mean you are more likely to drop them.

One of the most common injuries in gyms is weights dropped on feet. You've been warned!

 06 Make sure you are well hydrated before you start and that you keep a drink of water to hand while you are exercising. It's really important that you stay well hydrated as you'll be working hard.

 07 Always maintain good technique. If you can, exercise in front of a mirror to check your form when lifting.

 08 Breathe. It's something that sounds so simple and that we routinely do every second of our lives, yet I often have to remind my clients to continue to perform this fundamental action when they are exercise. Rhythmic breathing will help you to work more effectively too.

 09 The workouts in the programme are designed to be challenging. You will sweat and you will feel tired – but you should never feel as if you have pushed yourself to the point of feeling faint or unwell. Stop as soon as you do.

10 If you experience squeezing pressure in the chest, extreme shortness of breath, profuse sweating or no sweating, intense pain, nausea, and a red, hot appearance, your workout should be stopped and you should seek medical attention immediately.

Gym Equipment

Joining a gym is highly recommended for my 8-week plan. Many of the exercises I recommend involve basic equipment that you are unlikely to have at home

It's strongly advised that you use a local gym for the duration of this programme. You will need access to a range of equipment, some of which you might have at home, but not all. Gyms can be extremely reasonable and you certainly do not need to pay over the odds for swanky surroundings. Indeed, some research has shown that people work harder in more primitive gym surroundings as there is less to distract them from their training efforts.

Make sure your gym has most of the following:

Incline bench: An adjustable gym bench is used for many of the exercises in the book.

Dumbbells: These weights are essential as they will help to bring muscle tension and definition. You will likely need access to a variety of weights as you get stronger and fitter.

Barbell: This is a long metal bar to which discs of varying weights are attached at each end.

Treadmill: Not everyone likes running and you certainly won't be doing a lot of it on this programme. But access to a treadmill will add variety to your routines and I have included some treadmill work in my Finisher routines (see page 128).

VersaClimber: Most gyms will have this piece of equipment installed. It works all of the major muscle groups – arms, chest, shoulders, back, glutes, hips and legs – in a climbing motion to provide a low-impact workout. Great if you have issues with running or cycling.

Box or platform: These are usually simple wooden boxes that can be made higher or lower depending on your experience and strength. My advice is to start at the lowest height and master the technique before adding more height.

Kettlebells: Start with a bell weighing 16kg and gradually progress up to weights of 20-25kg per bell. If you are buying some bells for home use, remember there's more to them than weight – think about the handle. If it is rough or has seams, it could cause blisters. And also check it fits your hands. You can get small bells of a heavy weight and larger bells of a lighter weight.

Exercise bike: A gym staple, so you should have no problem finding one of these to use. A common mistake is to position the saddle wrongly, so really make sure it's set up for you before you start.

Indoor rower: Concept 2 rowers are the gold standard, but there are many other brands in gyms that are more than adequate. Make sure you get someone to check your technique. Poor rowing form is asking for niggles and injuries in the long term. Aiming to make the stroke longer and slower is far more effective than pulling too hard and fast. The whole stroke should blend as a continuous flow. And the action comes from the legs, not the arms.

Home Equipment

You don't need to clutter your home with lots of gym accessories, but some investment is worthwhile. I suggest trying the following (which can be purchased cheaply)

Heart rate monitor: Not essential, but very useful if you want to keep tabs on your heart rate variability (see page 82) and also to check your fitness progress. Again there is a huge variety of options – from chest strap HRMs (considered the most accurate) to wrist-worn, which are improving in terms of the technology and accuracy they provide.

Foam roller: These are extremely useful for soft tissue release. They come in a variety of sizes and levels of firmness. If you haven't used one before, try buying a medium density roller to begin with. Those with small circular bumps can help stimulate lymphatic drainage and boost circulation.

Exercise or yoga mat: I recommend stretching daily, even when you are not at the gym, so a slightly cushioned and non-slip exercise mat is a useful purchase.

A decent pair of trainers: There are trainers for everything and you could spend a small fortune purchasing shoes for every type of exercise – but it's not necessary. Visit a specialist sports shop and ask for advice, but if in doubt opt for a good, supportive running shoe. For many of the gym routines I would advocate not having much of a supportive shoe at all. The minimal the support, the better and the more control on the floor you have with the feet. This connection with the floor strengthens the foot and trains more control into the body. Check out Vivo-Barefoot shoes or other minimal training shoes.

Comfortable workout clothing: You can spend anything from £10 to £200 on a performance tee-shirt, so what you wear depends largely on your budget. Of prime importance is comfort. Make sure the fabric is lightweight and seamfree, that it has some sweat-wicking properties and that it fits well – you'd be amazed how many clients I see in expensive but ill-fitting gym clothing. Don't forget socks, which need to be comfortable and seamfree – they are often overlooked and inferior socks can cause blisters.

Matt Says:

All you need to embark on your fitness programme are some basic at-home essentials that won't cost the earth

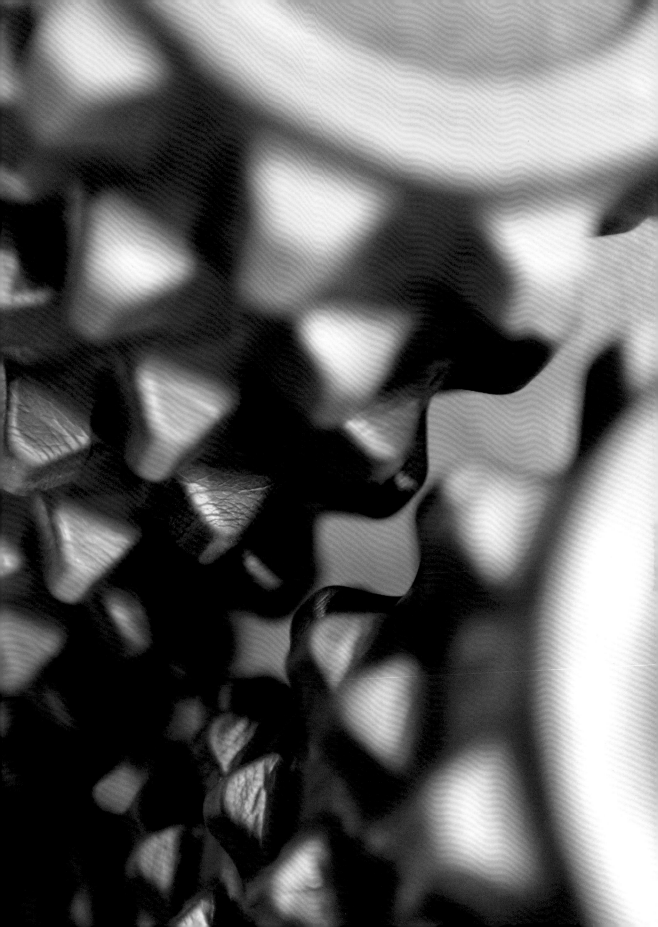

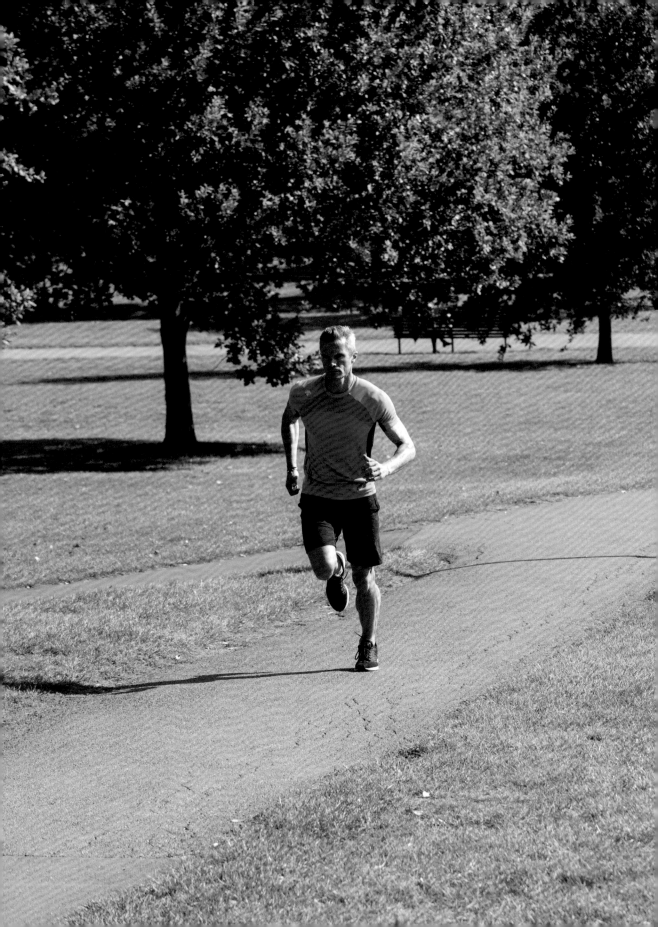

Chapter Nine

Exercises

Correct form and technique is of prime importance with any exercise plan, especially if you are attempting moves that you have never tried before. I can't stress enough how important it is to get this right and would advise you to practise moves in front of a mirror or accompanied by a partner at first, to make sure you get them spot on.

Everyday Stretches

Mobility and flexibility are hugely important, but often overlooked, aspects of fitness. They matter because they enable us to move more freely and to avoid the postural problems that inhibit our fitness progress. As we get older, our flexibility declines by quite a rapid rate, but we can stem that deterioration with regular stretching. I'm not saying that you need to do all of these stretches every day. But by incorporating them into your routine – make them a habit when you are sitting in front of the TV, for example – you will reap the benefits.

90/90 Hip Stretch

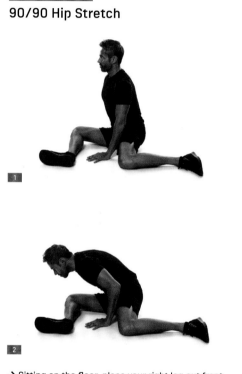

→ Sitting on the floor, place your right leg out front. Bend your knee at 90 degrees so your outer thigh and outer lower leg are resting on the floor. Your thigh should be perpendicular to your body. Place your other leg out to the side with the inner thigh touching the floor and the knee bent at 90 degrees. Place your hands on the floor on each side of the front leg. Slowly lower your chest towards your knee, keeping your shoulders squared to the floor. Don't drop to the elbow unless both can be on the floor equally. With this stretch even just sitting in the initial position and moving around a little will really help mobilise your hips.

Cobra to Child's Pose

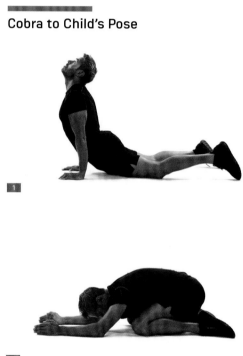

→ Lie face down on the floor with your hands underneath your shoulders, fingers pointing forwards. Lift your chest away from the floor by pressing your palms into the ground, keeping your elbows close to your body. Your elbows should be positioned directly under your shoulders. Hold this stretch for 4-5 seconds. To transition to Child's Pose, lift your hips off the ground, keeping your knees and forearms on the floor, and sit backward until your bottom rests on your heels. Let your forehead come close to the floor. Hold this position for 4-5 seconds.

Downward Dog

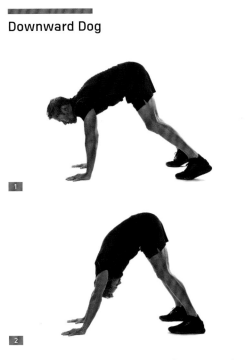

1

2

→ Start on your hands and knees, making sure your hands are directly underneath your shoulders, with fingers pointing forwards, and your knees directly underneath your hips. As you exhale, lift and straighten your knees, without locking them. Bring your body into the shape of an 'A', lifting through your pelvis. As you lengthen your spine, lift your sit bones up toward the ceiling, pressing down through your heels and palms of your hands. Relax your head, but do not let it dangle. Focus between your legs or towards your navel and hold for as long as is comfortable.

Side-lying Windmill

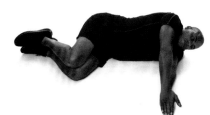

1

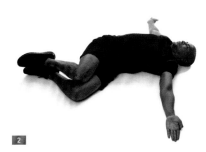

2

→ Lie on your left side with your knees bent and stacked on top of each other. Keep your left shoulder and hip rooted to the ground. Bring both of your arms straight out to your left side. Your arms should stack on top of each other. Rotate the right arm up and over your head while trying to touch your fingers to the ground. Allow your eyes to follow your arm for as long as possible. Rotate fully around to the starting position. Pause briefly and start again.

Couch Stretch

→ With your back to a bench or couch, kneel in front of it. Place your left foot up onto the edge or top of the couch behind you. The left knee should be close to the bottom of the bench or couch. Then place your right foot forward so your knee is bent at 90 degrees and gradually raise your body, by first moving your hands on to your front thigh and then lifting the chest up tall. While doing this also try to push the hip of the bent back knee forward to increase the stretch in the top of the thigh and hip. You will find the stretch varies day-to-day depending on what you have been doing. On days where you have sat for long periods it will feel harder, showing how tight your body is. Relax into this stretch and really try to develop it. It can be particularly helpful for back problems, so practise regularly.

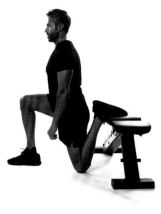

Pre-workout Mobility Drills

To get the most out of your workouts, it's important to make sure you are fully prepared for action. These mobility exercises will ensure that the body parts you are using are ready for the work that lies ahead.

Adductor Mobiliser

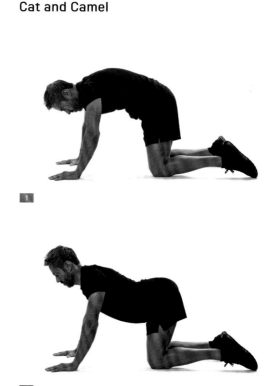

1

2

→ Start on all fours, then take one leg straight out to your side as far from the body as you can get. From this position place your elbows and forearms on the floor and then push your bottom back towards the heel behind you. Keep your leg straight and as you move back you should feel the stretch in your inner thigh and groin area. Repeat on the other side.

Cat and Camel

1

2

→ Start on all fours, with knees hip-width apart and your hands directly beneath your shoulders. Arch your back up towards the ceiling. Hold for 10 seconds, then slowly relax your back. Allow your stomach to drop toward the floor and lift your head slightly. Hold for 10 seconds, then return to the starting position.

TIP: When rounding your back, be conscious of tucking your pelvis under in order to encourage a fuller range of motion

Couch Stretch with Reach

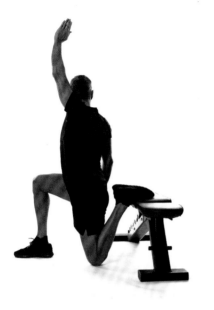

→ With your back to a bench or couch, kneel in front of it. Place one foot up onto the edge or top of the couch behind you. The knee of that foot should be close to the bottom of the bench or couch. Then place your other foot forward so your knee is bent at 90 degrees and gradually bring your body up by first moving your hands on to your front thigh and then lifting the chest up tall. While doing this also try to push the hip of the bent back knee forward to increase the stretch in the top of the thigh and hip. Then lift the arm of the leg that is behind high up into the air to increase the stretch across the hip. Repeat on the other side.

Reach Through

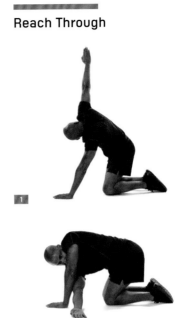

→ Start on all fours with knees hip-width apart and your hands directly beneath your shoulders. Inhale and allow your right hand to lift up off the mat, and rotate up toward the ceiling, opening your chest to the right. Look up towards your fingers. Pause then exhale and bring your right hand down crossing under your body, feeding through the gap between your left arm and left knee. This will bring your right shoulder, arm and ear close to the floor. Inhale and repeat. Repeat on the other side.

Kneeling Hip Flexors

→ Start by kneeling on the floor. Lift up your right knee and place your right foot on the floor in front of you so that your right knee is directly over your right ankle. Place both hands on your right thigh to help maintain a tall spine. Lean forward into your right hip while keeping your left knee pressed into the floor. Repeat on the other side.

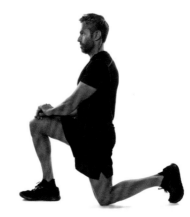

Pre-workout Activation Drills

In addition to mobility, we need to make sure that the muscles you are using are primed – or activated – for the workload that I am prescribing. That's where these drills come in. They essentially 'fire up' the large muscles that will be working hardest in the exercise routines that follow.

Banded Pull Apart

→ Stand with feet shoulder-width apart. Hold an exercise band in both hands in front of you at about chest height and pull it apart by squeezing your shoulder blades together and stretching your arms out to the sides. Bring both arms back together in a controlled way and repeat.

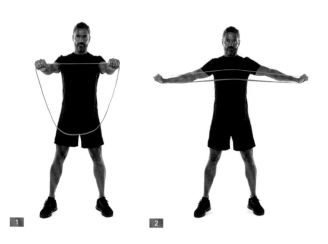

Bird Dog

→ Start on all fours with knees hip-width apart and your hands directly beneath your shoulders. Extend and straighten your right leg out behind you until it is nearly parallel to the floor. Stretch your left arm out in front of you, keeping your neck aligned with your spine. Gently lower yourself back to the starting position. Repeat with the opposite limbs.

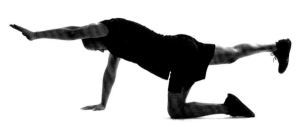

Clam

→ Lie on your right side with your legs stacked on top of each other. Rest your head on your bent bottom arm. Bend your top arm and anchor your left thumb just below the waist. Keeping your heels together, slowly rotate your leg in the hip socket to open your knees like a clamshell. Don't allow yourself to wobble off balance. Open your knee only as far as you can go without disturbing the alignment of your hips. Slowly bring your knee back to the start position. Repeat 3 to 5 times on one side before changing sides.

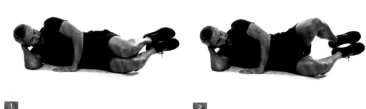

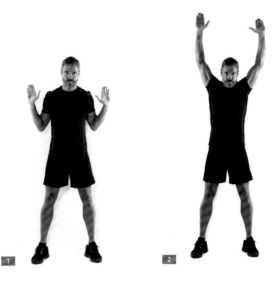

Wall Angel

→ Stand with your back to a wall. With your arms flat against the wall, bend your elbows with your forearms and hands pointing upwards. Your heels would be as close to the wall as possible with your hips and spine pressed into the wall. Begin to straighten your arms directly overhead, trying to keep the elbows sliding up against the wall as far as you can - up to the height of your ears and back down to your lower ribs. Repeat.

Glute Bridge

→ Lie on your back with knees bent and feet flat on the floor hip-width apart. Exhale and lift your hips upwards so your back lifts off the floor. Inhale and slowly lower yourself back into the starting position.

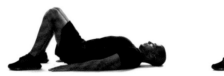

Lateral Banded Walk

→ Stand with your feet shoulder-width apart. Place an exercise band under your feet and hold the other end in your hands in front of you at chest height. Bend your knees so you are in a half-squat position. Make sure you stay evenly balanced and 'walk' forward with small steps for approximately 6-8 short 'strides'. Return and repeat.

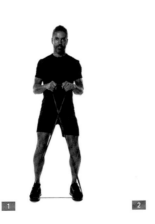
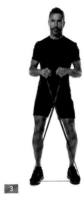

Main Workout Exercises

These exercises make up the main part of each of your workout days. Take the time to read the instructions thoroughly and to really understand each part of each movement. That way, as we load up the movements, you'll achieve the maximum result with the lowest risk of injury.

Alternating Spiderman

→ Start in the raised plank position with hands on the floor shoulder-width apart and arms extended, toes gripping the floor and hip-width apart. Make sure your core is engaged. Bring your left foot up to the outside of your left hand, trying to maintain as straight a back as possible by raising your chest as you step forward. Return to the start position and repeat with the right foot.

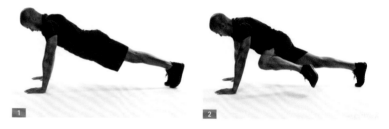

Bench Press

→ Lie on your back on a bench with your feet flat on the floor and knees bent. Hold a barbell with your hands just wider than shoulder-width apart. Slowly lower the bar to your chest, keeping a strong position across the shoulder blades and the elbows slightly squeezed down to keep tension out of the trapezius muscles. Now return to the start position with a strong press action. Repeat.

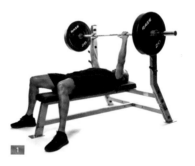
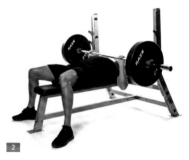

Bent Over Row

→ Stand with feet shoulder-width apart. Hold a barbell with hands shoulder-width apart and palms down. Bend forwards, hingeing forward from your hips. Bend your knees and keep your back straight. Your arms should hang straight down. Now squeeze your shoulders together to row the barbell up towards your chest. Then slowly lower the bar to the starting position and repeat.

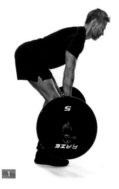
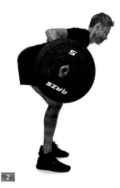

Bicep Curl

→ Hold a dumbbell in each hand. Stand with your legs hip-width apart and your palms facing outwards. Keep a neutral spine and your knees slightly flexed. Curl the weights up to your chest by bending your elbows. Keep your elbows tucked into the sides of your body. Lower the dumbbells back to the start position by straightening your arms slowly. Repeat.

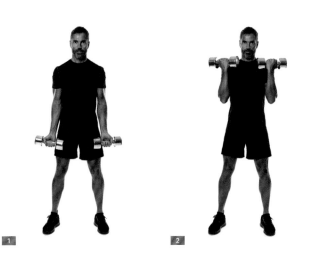

Burpee

→ Begin in a crouched position on your toes with hands touching the floor beside your feet and knees tucked into the body. Kick your feet straight out behind you and jump them back in again to the starting position. Come into a standing position by leaping into the air with both arms raised overhead. Return again to the starting position and repeat.

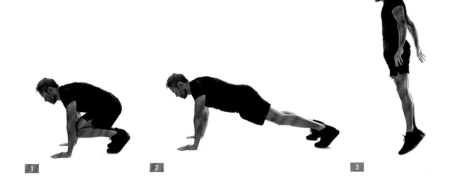

Double Kettlebell Straight Leg Deadlift

→ Place two kettlebells between your feet with the handles lined up. Bend your knees and hinge forward at the hips to grab the handles of the kettlebells. Now stand up straight, roll your shoulders back and completely flatten out your back. Hinge forwards from your waist, keeping your legs straight and stiff to lower the kettlebell towards the floor. Pause at the bottom of the movement, avoiding any bounce, before returning to the starting position.

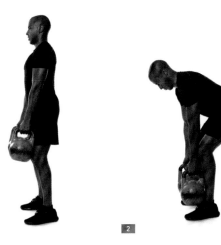

Dumbbell Chest Press

→ Lie on your back on a flat bench with feet hip-width apart on the floor and a dumbbell in each hand. Squeeze your glutes tight to hold the pelvis in place. In the bracing position, take the dumbbells out to your side but angled slightly up towards the top of your body. Then squeeze the shoulder blades back and make sure that the chest is pushed forward. Now, keeping your shoulders back, push the dumbbells up above your mid chest point. The emphasis of the movement is in the chest muscles. Lower under control and repeat.

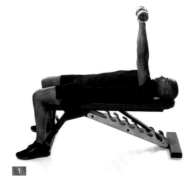
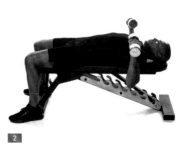

Dumbbell Pullover

→ Lie on your back on a flat bench with feet on the floor, weight balanced on your heels. Hold a single dumbbell in both hands and position over your chest with arms extended. Lower the dumbbell behind your head keeping your arms fairly straight. Make sure your back stays as flat to the bench as possible. Return to the starting position.

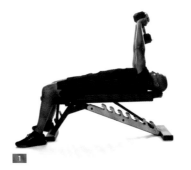
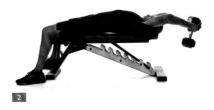

Face Pull

→ Use a high pulley with a rope or dual handles. Stand with feet shoulder-width apart and knees slightly bent. Hold the handle in an overhand grip (palms facing downwards) with your arms fully extended out in front of you. At this point, you should be able to feel your shoulder blades being slightly pulled out. Pull the handles towards your face, separating your hands so the handles go either side of your face and squeezing your shoulder blades back into a tight squeezed central position. Then slowly return to the starting position.

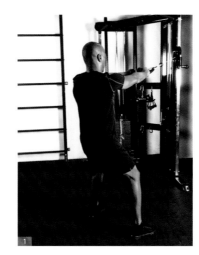
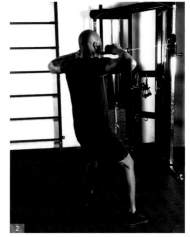

Hammer Curl

→ Sit on an upright exercise bench in a slightly inclined position. Hold a dumbbell in each hand with your arms hanging down by your side in a straight line. Your thumbs should be facing forwards. Keeping your elbows close to your body, curl the dumbbells up towards your shoulders. Now slowly lower the dumbbells back to the starting point

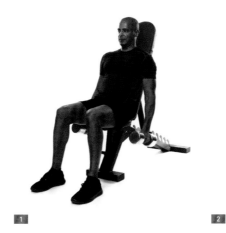 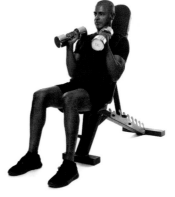

Incline Dumbbell Press

→ Lie on an incline bench with your feet flat on the floor and a dumbbell in each hand. Hold the dumbbells to the side of your chest with palms facing forward, your elbows bent at a 90-degree angle and your shoulders pulled down and back. Now press the dumbbells up over your head with your elbows fully extended. Don't bend at the wrists. Slowly lower the dumbbells back down towards your chest, but moving slightly wider towards the armpits. Repeat.

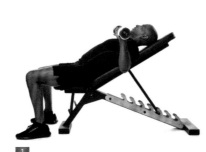 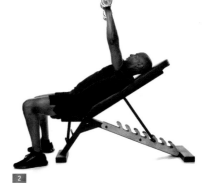

Kettlebell Rack-position Squat

→ Stand with your feet slightly angled out and wider than shoulder-width apart. Clasp your fingers together and lift the kettlebells to rest them on the front of your shoulders or upper arms. Simultaneously hinge the knees and hips, aiming to sit between your heels in a squat position. Aim for a slight forward lean in your torso but keep your chest up and don't allow your upper body to collapse forward. Keep your back straight. As you stand up and return to the starting position, press your body away from the floor by squeezing your glutes, quads and hamstrings. As you reach the top position, extend your knees by squeezing your quads and hamstrings. Don't allow your knees to collapse in or fall outwards.

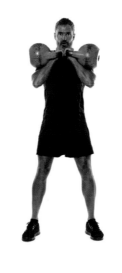 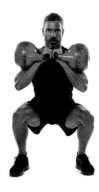

Kettlebell Single Leg Deadlift

→ Stand with feet hip-width apart holding a kettlebell in each hand. Now hinge forward as you almost lock your left knee and raise your right leg behind you. Go as far down as you can comfortably go – you should feel a stretch in your hamstrings at the backs of your legs – lowering your dumbbells in the process. Keep your back completely flat and squeeze your shoulder blades together.

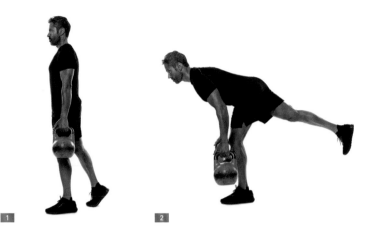

Lat Pull Down

→ Sit on the lat pull down machine and adjust the knee pad so that there is no free space and you are tightly seated. Place your feet flat on the floor and push your chest upwards and out. Extend your arms up and take hold of the bar with your hands in a wide grip (this should be on the declined portion of the long bar, both sides). When you're in this starting position, inhale, making sure you don't let your scapula loosen or your shoulders raise. Exhale when you begin the movement. Pull down the bar in front of you through your elbows until you're able to squeeze your lats at the bottom of the movement and your shoulder blades are together. Slowly raise the bar back up until your arms are extended and back in the starting position.

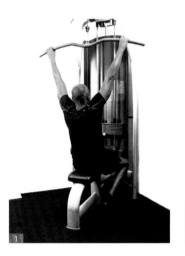
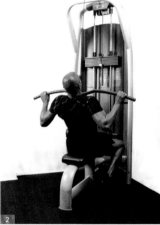

Lateral Lunge

→ Stand with feet shoulder-width apart holding a dumbbell in a goblet fashion. Take a stride out to your right, lowering your bottom towards the floor on that side as if going to sit down. Extend your left leg so it is straight and keep your chest up. Make sure that as you lower your bodyweight the control is coming from the glutes on the striding side. Then push up through the hip and come back up to standing.

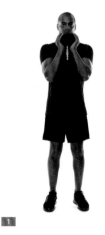
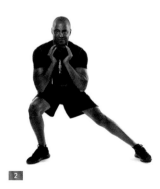

Lateral Lunge with Heel Touch

→ Stand with your feet together, then take a stride out towards your left side, controlling the stride with the thigh and glutes of your moving leg. Now bring your right hand down to touch the inside of the opposite ankle before powerfully pushing back up to your starting position. Repeat on the other side.

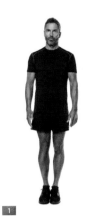
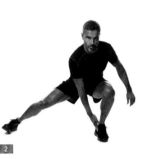

Lateral Raise

→ Stand with feet shoulder-width apart, arms straight at the sides, holding a dumbbell in each hand. Have a slight bend in your knees and elbows. Slowly raise both arms outwards until your hands are level with your shoulders. Hold at this top position for a second. Lower your arms to the starting position and repeat.

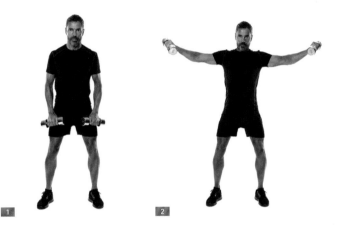

Mountain Climber

→ Start in a strong press-up position with hands shoulder-width apart. Keep your shoulders firmly in position, your core muscles engaged and legs straight. There should be a strong straight line through the body. Now draw one knee up in towards your chest while keeping the rest of the body very straight, then return it to the start position and repeat on the other side. Maintain an even tempo and hold your body straight throughout.

TIP: Technique, technique, technique. How you perform each and every exercise is vital to success

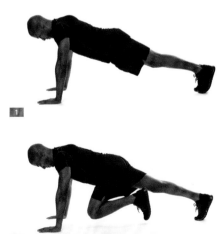

Press-up

→ Start in the raised plank position with hands on the floor shoulder-width apart and arms extended, toes gripping the floor and hip-width apart. Maintain a straight line through the body by keeping the muscles through the core tight at all times. Whilst in the top position of the press-up, gently pull the shoulder blades back so you are aware of them with the chest positioned forward. Maintain this positioning throughout the movement. Now, bending your elbows, lower your body down towards the floor, maintaining a straight line and keeping tension in the arms. Then, in a controlled fashion, push your back up so your arms are extended.

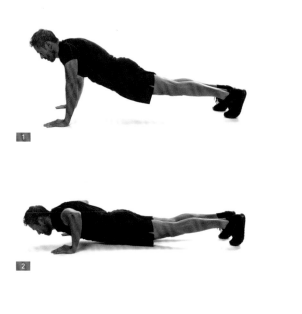

Nordic Curl

→ You can do this exercise on a machine, with feet tucked under a heavy piece of equipment or with a partner holding your ankles. Kneel on the ground, with someone sitting behind you to hold your ankles. As slowly and smoothly as possible, lean forward so that your chest approaches the ground. Use your hamstrings to control your forward momentum until you can no longer resist gravity. Put out your arms at that time to halt your fall. When your chest touches the ground, push yourself upright to the start position.

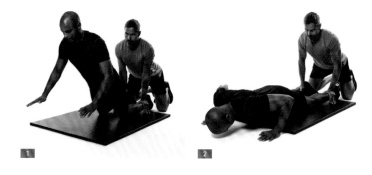

→ Nordic Curls

Did you know that plenty of recent studies suggest that almost two-thirds of hamstring injuries could be prevented if Nordic Curls were practised on a regular basis? One trial [1] involving Danish footballers assigned participants to either a programme that focused heavily on the hamstring curl or one of normal strength training (not including the Nordic move). During the season that followed, those who had practised the Nordic Curl experienced 70 per cent fewer injuries than the control group. Among players who had previously suffered hamstring problems, the injury rate dropped by 85 per cent. Another study published by the American College of Sports Medicine [2] analysed the hamstring muscle fibre lengths of 28 healthy men before asking them to embark on either a six-week training schedule of moves with lengthening muscle contractions – including the Nordic curl – or a programme of shortening contractions. Previous trials had suggested that shorter muscle fibres increase the risk of hamstring injury in elite athletes and this was no different.

Raised Plank with Forward Reach

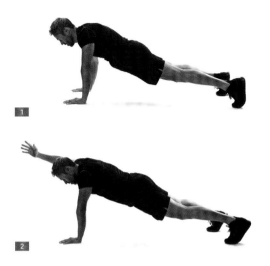

→ Start in the raised plank position with hands on the floor shoulder-width apart and arms extended, toes gripping the floor and hip-width apart. Your body should form a straight line from your shoulders to your heels. Then reach forward with one arm, holding for a couple of seconds. Return to starting position and reach forward with the other arm.

Raised Plank with Shoulder Touch

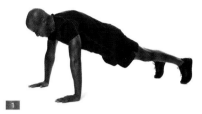

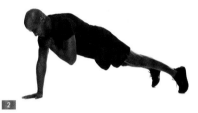

→ Start in the raised plank position with hands on the floor shoulder-width apart and arms extended, toes gripping the floor and hip-width apart. Maintain a straight line through the body with your hips held firm. Keep your weight distributed between your arms and feet and brace the mid-section. Holding this position, take your left hand off the floor and touch your opposite shoulder. Place your hand back on the floor and repeat on the other side. Whilst performing this alternating movement, aim to keep the body still and prevent any rolling through the hips.

Raised Press-up

→ Lie on the floor face down and place your hands about shoulder-width apart with arms extended. Place your toes on top of a flat bench to elevate your body. The higher the elevation of the flat bench, the higher the resistance of the exercise is. Lower yourself by bending your arms until your chest almost touches the floor as you inhale. Use your pectoral muscles and arms to press your upper body back up to the starting position.

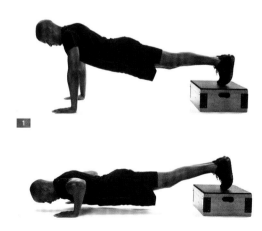

Pull-up

→ Stand under a chin-up bar and jump up to grip the bar firmly with hands shoulder-width apart. Hang with your arms fully extended. Keep your shoulders squeezed back and down. Slowly pull your body upwards by pulling your elbows down to your sides so your chin is above your hands. Pause at the top then slowly return to the starting position.

TIP: If at first you can't perform a full bodyweight pull-up, try using an assisted dip/chin machine if available at your gym

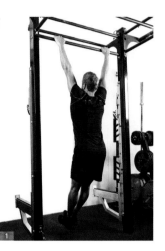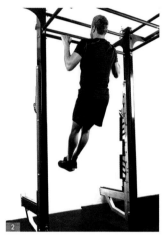

Reverse Fly

→ Standing with feet shoulder-width apart, hold a weight in each hand. Hinge forward to a 45-degree angle, maintaining a flat back. Keep knees lightly flexed. Without locking your elbows, raise your arms out to your side by concentrating the effort in the middle of the back. Slowly return to the starting position, being careful not to 'shrug' the weight. It should be a smooth return.

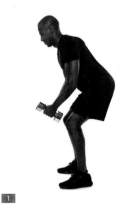

Rowing

→ This is perhaps the exercise technique that most people get wrong and, if you do, it can play havoc with your back and shoulders. What a lot of people don't realise is that the power of rowing comes from the legs, and the initial drive phase begins with a powerful push from the legs. Drive until your legs are almost fully extended and the hips begin to open up. At full extension of the legs, make sure your back is vertical, and start to bring the handle in towards the body with your arms. Keep the line of the handle and your wrists to stay in line with your forearms. Bring in towards the chest until your legs and back straighten. Next is the recovery phase - basically the drive phase in reverse. Begin by straightening the arms. Then pivot your body from the hips before bending your legs until your shins are vertical. Throughout the movement, keep your back flat, pivoting from the hips. Once back at the start position, repeat with fluid and rhythmical motion.

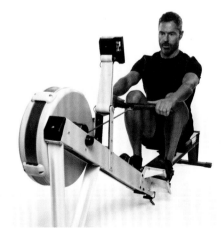

Seated Cable Row

→ Using a cable machine, start in a seated position with feet flat on the floor and knees bent. Hold the bar in both hands with your arms stretched out in front of you. Now maintaining a strong bracing position, pull the bar towards your belly button, keeping your body in the same position and concentrating on pulling your elbows back and into your ribs.

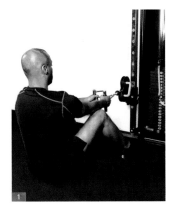
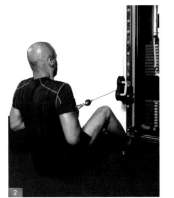

Shoulder Press

→ Sit on an upright exercise bench with your feet hip-width apart. Keep your back straight, abdominal muscles engaged and knees bent. Your chest muscles should be relaxed. Hold a dumbbell in each hand and, bending your elbows, position them out to the side of your shoulders with palms facing forwards. Press the dumbbell to extend upwards to above your head and then slowly lower back to the starting position. Keep your shoulder blades down and back to prevent the shoulders creeping forward.

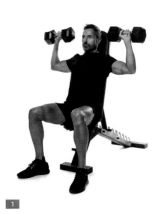
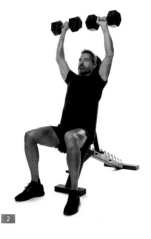

Single Arm Row

→ Hold a weight in your right hand. Put your left knee and left hand on a bench keeping your right foot on the floor to the side. With a flat back, allow your right arm to hang straight down and level with the shoulder. At this point make sure you have activated the muscles of the upper back. Lift the weight until it is level with your back, keeping your arm close to your side, squeezing your shoulder blades and tucking the weight into your rib cage. Lower the weight back to the starting position.

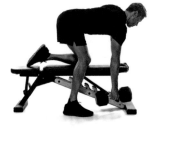

Trap Bar Deadlift

→ The Trap Bar is an unusual looking bar, but with its neutral grip and a less complex moving pattern than the conventional deadlift, it allows quicker strength and power development for the user.

Stand in the centre of the bar with feet hip-width apart with knees flexed, then place your hands in the middle of the grips so that your hands are to the side of your knees. Now straighten your back and push your bottom outwards. Squeeze the muscle in your bottom, brace your mid-section, grip the bar and pull your shoulder blades back. Keep your chin in a neutral position and upper back muscles strong at all times. Then push forward with the hips and allow that movement to naturally straighten the body up. At the top of the movement, the muscles in the bottom should be working hard and the hips should be forward. Your shoulder and upper back muscles should be holding your shoulders back with your chest pushed forward. Now lower yourself back down to the starting position. It is really important that the brace is held at the top of the movement and then into the lowering phase.

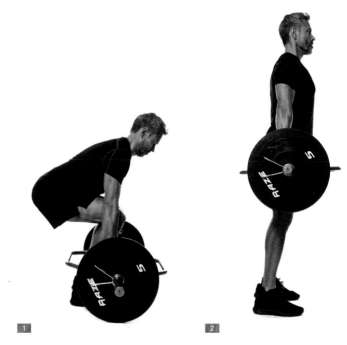

1

2

→ Bracing

One of the key elements to successfully getting stronger and being able to lift more weight in the gym is the way you set your body up before performing any movement. The 'bracing' or 'ready' position is essential to make the most of the work you put in. It is also essential to train the body to hold the spine in a better position during all activities.

To learn how to properly 'brace', first lie on the floor, with your knees bent up, placing your hands so your fingers are on the front of your tummy and your thumbs are in to the sides. Then practise using the muscles around your mid-section to push out against your fingers. The aim of this is not to breathe in to create the push, but instead to 'brace' with the muscles. It is also not just about pushing your tummy out; it is about trying to 'brace' the muscles at the front, back and to each side of the body. Once in this bracing position, you should be able to breathe freely and should not be holding your breath at all.

Now practise this position while standing up. Once you have mastered this position, it is the automatic position you should go in to before any strength movement you perform. Be it for a squat, a deadlift or a bench press, the bracing position will protect the body and make a stronger movement. Add to this the tensing of your grip muscles, your feet into the floor, your glutes and hips held tight and upper body muscles of the back and you are then ready to perform.

Single Leg Glute Bridge

→ Lie on your back and bend your knees so your feet rest flat on the floor. Raise one leg so that the knee comes up in line with the hip. Tuck the pelvis towards you slightly then push the body off the floor with the one leg still on the floor. Pull the belly button in and lead with the hip, by pushing through the bottom, while keeping the body very straight.

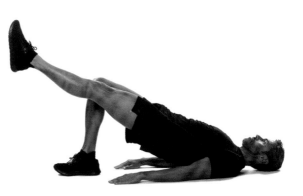

Squat Thrust

→ Place your hands on the floor shoulder-width apart with legs straight out behind your body. Make sure your body is in a straight line. Jump both legs in towards your chest as far as you can by bending at the knees. Return to the starting position by jumping your legs back.

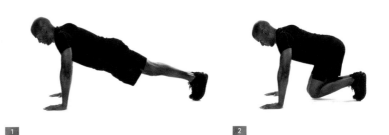

Single Leg Deadlift

→ Hold a weight in your right hand and engage your core for best posture. Standing on your right leg, lean forward and extend your right leg out behind you while maintaining a straight back, level hips and a slightly flexed left knee. Move as if hinged from the hips. Lower your upper body in a straight line, maintaining your position and keeping your right arm straight. Hold your left arm level with your upper body. Return to the start position, squeezing the glutes as you do.

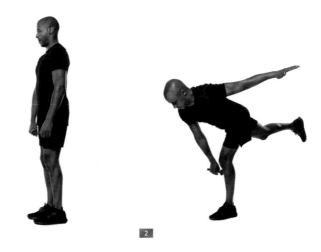

Squat

→ Stand with feet wider than shoulder-width apart and arms extended out in front of you. Bend from the hips and aim to keep your body weight pressed into your heels. Maintain a straight back. Bend your knees until they are almost at 90 degrees. Push back up to the start position and repeat.

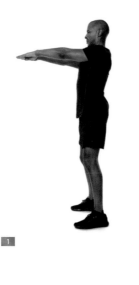

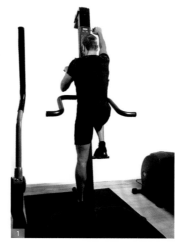

VersaClimber

→ Long overlooked as an exercise machine, the VersaClimber is coming into its own as trainers realise its value in offering a unique climbing action that incorporates the arms and legs. The machine is built at a 75-degree climb angle that reduces the isolated weight bearing on the knees, slightly unloading the lower back.

To use it, first step on the lower pedal and hold the lower handgrip. Repeat with the higher pedal and hold the higher grip. Begin by moving through the full range of motion of your arms and legs. As you 'climb', your opposite arm and leg with be extended. Continue alternating in this way.

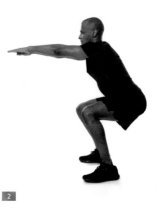

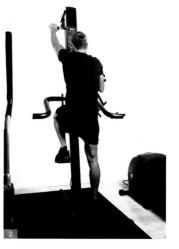

→ ## Did you know?

A study published in the journal *Medicine and Science in Sports and Exercise* [3] showed that training on the VersaClimber elicits a greater VO_2 max response – a measure of cardio effort – than running on a treadmill or using the indoor rower.

Triceps Push Down

→ Use a tricep rope attachment on a pulley machine. Stand with feet hip-width apart and knees slightly bent. Keeping your elbows close to your stomach and shoulders pinned back, grip the rope with a pronated grip (palms facing downwards) and shoulder-width apart. Leaning slightly forwards, push the rope down using only your triceps until the ends almost hit your upper thigh. At this point, the arms should be fully extended. Keep your shoulders and arms still throughout the movement so that only the forearms are moving. Squeeze your triceps for 1 to 2 seconds at this point of the move then slowly release the rope back to the starting position.

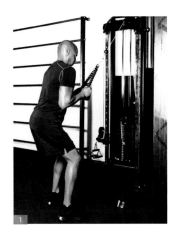 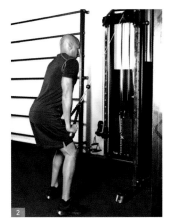

Walking Lunge

→ Holding a weight in each hand, stand with feet hip-width apart. Take a stride forward with your right leg and lower your body towards the floor, keeping your shoulders back and your chest up. Bend both knees to 90 degrees at the bottom of the movement so your right knee is above your right foot and your left knee below your hips. Now stride forward with your opposite leg. Repeat for the required number of strides.

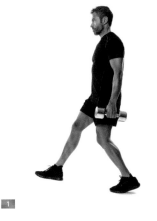 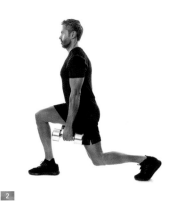

Weighted Split Squat

→ Start by placing a box, step or bench in front you. Hold a weight in each hand and take a stride forward with your right leg so that your foot is on the box. Your left foot should be flat on the floor. Bend your front knee so it is above your front shoe laces. Lower your back knee down towards the floor, while keeping the chest up and stomach muscles tight. Repeat on the other side.

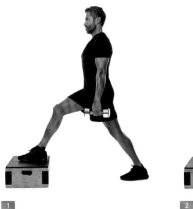 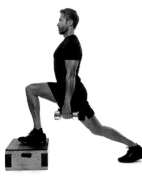

Post-workout Stretches

So many people neglect post-workout stretches and it really can hamper your progress. These exercises are designed to be performed when your muscles are warm (i.e. after a workout) so that you maximise the effect of the stretching process. By doing them, you will not only improve flexibility, but enhance your recovery process.

Band or Towel Hamstring Stretch

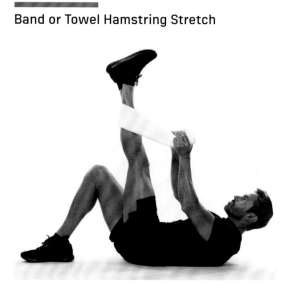

→ Lie on the floor on your back with your legs bent and feet flat on the floor. Loop an exercise band or towel around the back of your left calf. Raise your left leg by pulling the towel or band towards you while keeping the knee straight. Pull it until you feel a stretch in the hamstring and hold for up to 30 seconds. Lower back down and repeat on the other side.

TIP: For many of us, the hip flexors become very tight because we spend so much time seated. Stretching them regularly is essential

Hip Flexor Stretch

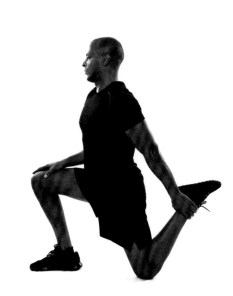

→ From a kneeling position, step one foot out in front of you. Then reach back and take hold of the lace area of your shoe. Keeping the hip pressed gently forward, bring the foot up behind you to feel the stretch in the quad and hip.

Banded or Hanging Back Stretch

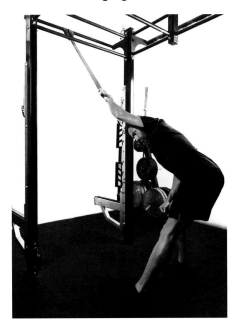

→ This stretch for the back can be done using a fitness band or just a wall bar. Either holding onto a wall bar or gripping the fitness band with one hand, allow the body to hang back and relax the muscles of the upper back. Then gradually drop the hip of the side you are stretching, away from the stretch point. You should feel a lovely stretch right down the side of the body.

Banded or Upright Pec Stretch

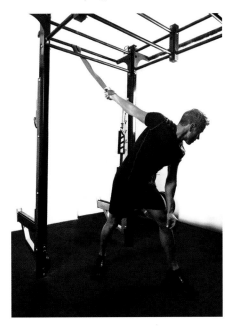

→ Either holding on to a fitness band or upright post, rotate the body away from the stretch point and feel the stretch across the chest. Perform this stretch on both sides.

Glute Stretch

→ Lie on your back with your knees bent. Lift your right ankle up and rest it across the left knee. Reach underneath the left leg and pull up towards your chest. Repeat with the opposite leg.

TIP: If you have difficulty reaching the thigh, use a towel looped around your thigh to enable the stretch

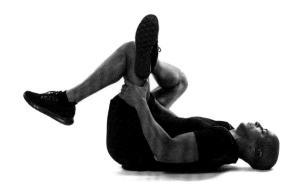

Soft Tissue Roller Work

Stretching and mobility work helps to keep things supple and mobile, but we also need to release fascia, the dense, fibrous connective tissue around the body that encompasses all muscles and bones. In small amounts, fascia is protective, but when it builds up through bad habits, heavy workouts and injury it becomes restrictive, limiting our ability to move freely. Ignoring knots – or, to give them their medical term, myofascial adhesions – can worsen the dysfunction and potentially raise the risk of injury. This is where foam rollers come in as they can help break down these knots. I'm a big fan of rollers and recommend that most of my clients use one. They can be very inexpensive and are a great addition to your fitness kit cupboard.

Adductors

→ Lie on your front with one leg out to the side and the foot turned outwards. Place the roller under your mid-inner thigh on that leg and then roll along the inner thigh.

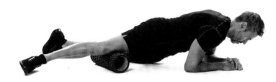

Calf Muscles

→ Sit down with your legs extended out in front of you. Place the roller at the mid-point of one calf and then place your other leg on top. Then roll over the roller going down from the mid-point and, once you have been up and down a few times, roll your foot to the side. Then roll again up and down the outside of your calf. Once you've done this a few times, turn your foot to the inside and roll up and down the inner line of your calf.

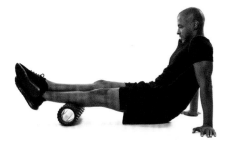

Glutes

→ Sitting on the roller, place one foot over the other knee and then lean towards the bent leg. With the roller pressing on the buttock, work up and down in a straight line across the buttock and hip area.

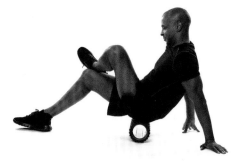

Hips

→ Lying on your front, try to work the roller under the bony section of the hip and slightly behind, right in to the top of the buttock.

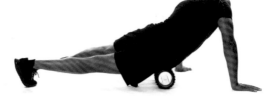

Ilio Tibial Band (ITB)

→ The ITB is a long tendinous band that goes from the hip down to the outside of the knee and its job is to help keep the knee straight. Depending on how we move or the amount of exercise we do and type of exercise we do, this tendon can get very tight. Once tight it can cause severe pain at the knee. Regular soft tissue work in this area will prevent this and also take pressure off the knee joint.

Lie on your side with the roller half-way down your thigh and gradually work your way up and down the outside of your leg.

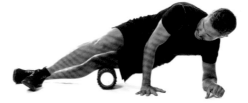

Lats

→ Lie on the floor with your body at 45 degrees. Place the roller under your arm and to the top of the upper back. Lift your bottom off the floor to place pressure on to the roller. Then roll up and down the lat muscle.

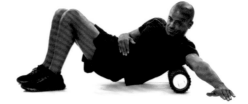

Quads

→ Lying on your front, start with the roller at the front of your mid-thigh and then move up and down the outside of your leg. Working in small movements, do this anywhere that feels particularly tight.

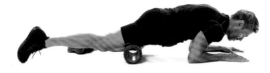

T-spine Release

→ Lie on your back and place the roller just under your shoulder blades. Keep your bottom on the floor and bring your hands up to the side of your temple with elbows out to the side. From here roll back over the roller, making sure to keep your chin in and your abdominal muscles tight so that the lumbar spine doesn't end up doing most of the work. The aim of this movement is to open up the upper back, not just see how far you can move.

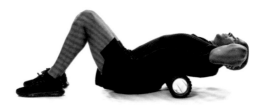

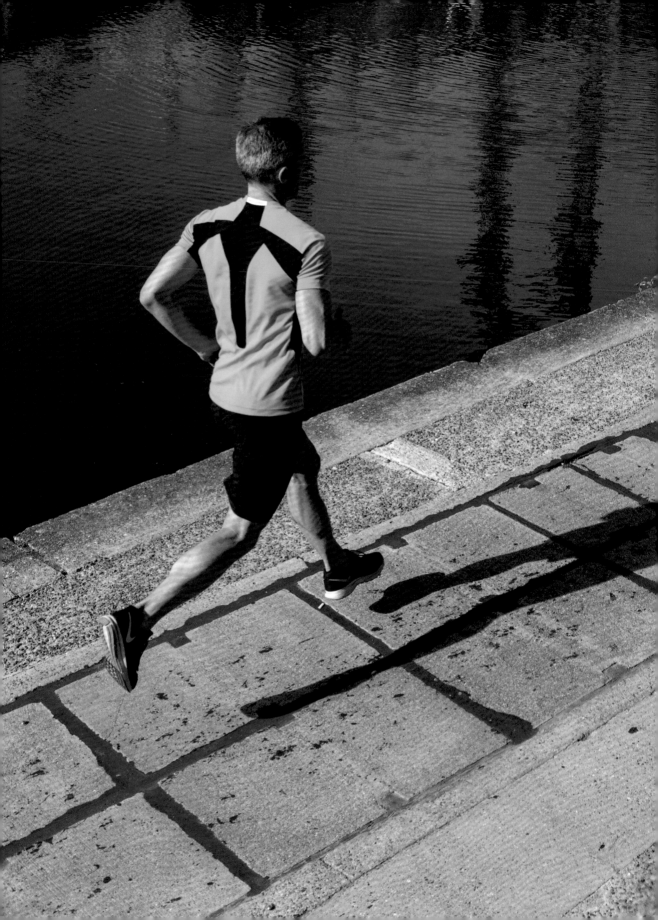

The Finishers

These mini workouts can be performed at the end of a session. The muscles targeted in these mini routines will already be worked during the regular workouts you are doing, but I just want to give you the option of a little more work.

You will see that there are instructions to include a finisher routine within the exercise programme. You can select from one of the routines in this chapter, choosing the one that is most relevant to your environment and circumstances.

Finisher Routine 1

My aim is to help you develop overall body strength. However, you may have a specific area that you want to improve and that requires some more targeted and intensive conditioning. That's where the Finishers come in. Perform each set for the stated number of reps, then move on to the next exercise. Continue until you've completed all the sets.

Kettlebell Swing

1	25 reps
2	20 reps
3	15 reps

→ Stand with feet shoulder-width apart and knees slightly bent. Place a kettlebell on the floor in front of your feet. Hinge forward at your hips to lean down and grip the kettlebell with both hands in a palms-down grip. Keep your shins vertical to the floor and your spine straight as you pull the kettlebell back between your legs. Push your hips forward and pull your knees back to generate the forward momentum to swing the kettlebell forward and up in front of your body. Strength should come from your legs and hips, not your shoulders. As the kettlebell reaches the top of the move, brace your abdominal muscles and contract your arm and shoulder muscles to create a brief pause before pulling the kettlebell back down between your legs for the next repetition.

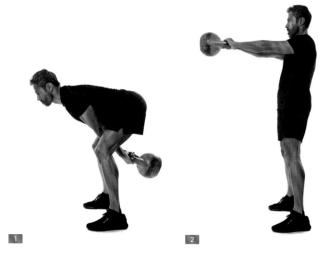

Russian Twist

1	20 reps
2	20 reps
3	20 reps

→ Sit on the floor with both knees slightly bent up and heels either off the floor or just touching without weight on the heels. Your back should be straight and a 'V' shape between the upper body and thighs. Holding a medicine ball or light kettlebell with both hands, move the weight from side to side. Whilst moving the weight across your body make sure that your shoulders move with the direction of the weight and keep your knees together at all times.

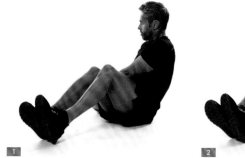
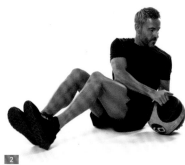

Raised Spiderman

1	15 reps
2	20 reps
3	25 reps

→ Place your forearms on a bench with shoulders placed over the elbows. With core muscles held tight, maintain a straight line through your body as if in the plank position. From this position pick your knee up and out to the side of your elbow squeezing the muscles in the outside of your hips to create the movement. Keep your foot off the floor throughout the movement and then return your foot back to the start position maintaining a strong posture throughout.

TIP: While not essential, the finishers can make a real difference to your overall progress, helping you to reach your desired end-goal

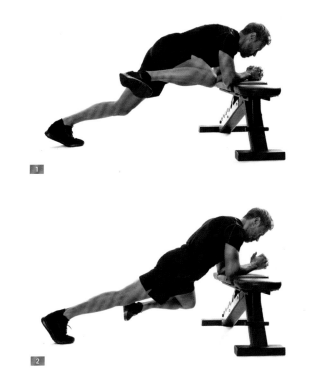

Sumo Deadlift

1	20 reps
2	20 reps
3	20 reps

→ Start with your feet wide apart and toes pointed out on the diagonal. Place two kettlebells between your feet. From this start position squat down, hingeing from the hips, to take hold of the kettlebells. Once in this position make sure the upper back muscles are strong and the shoulder blades are back. Maintaining this bracing at the core muscles and a strong hold in the upper back muscles, push the hips through so that the upper body rises up. Control the lowering phase, so that the kettlebells lower to the exact start position you started, and then repeat.

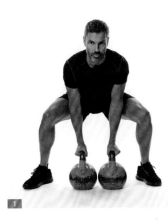

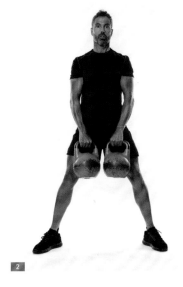

Finisher Routine 2

Cone Lunge

1	30 reps
2	30 reps
3	30 reps

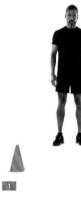

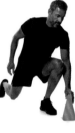

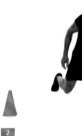

→ Set two cones on the floor out in front of you about 150-200cm apart. Standing back from the cones and in the middle, alternate lunges towards the cones while touching the cone with the same hand as the foot you lunge forward with. Right hand and foot to right side and left hand and foot to left side.

Bear Crawl

1	20 out 20 back
2	20 out 20 back
3	20 out 20 back

→ Start in a push-up position with hands shoulder-width apart and legs straight out directly behind your body about hip-width apart, keeping your knees bent. Push the toes of your right foot into the floor while squeezing your left thigh and glute. Move your right hand and left leg forward to start crawling. Alternate the arm and leg movements making sure to keep your back straight and hips and shoulders in line.

Walk Out Press-up

1	15 reps
2	15 reps
3	15 reps

→ Bend down into a deep squat position then place your hands on the floor in front of you. Walk your hands forward until your body is in a press-up position. Perform a press-up. Now walk your hands back to return to the deep squat position. Then stand up and repeat.

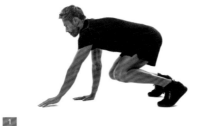

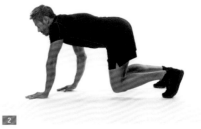

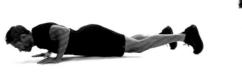

Hop Overs

1	30 reps
2	30 reps
3	30 reps

→ Start standing on top of a box (or bench) and then touch your feet down on the floor to one side of the box before hopping back on to the box and repeating on the other side. This should be done with speed and balance.

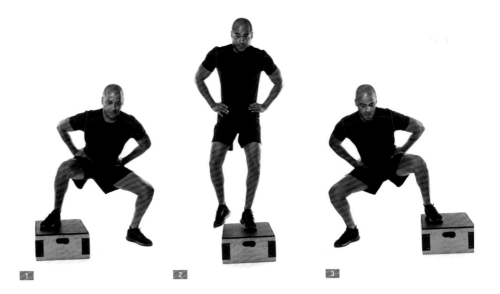

Finisher Routine 3

Versa Climber or Indoor Rowing Machine

1 | 2 mins
2 | 90 secs

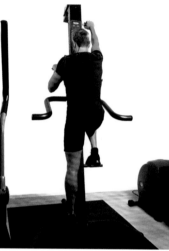

Treadmill Run

1 | 2 mins
2 | 90 secs

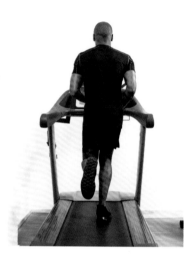

Indoor Bike

1 | 2 mins
2 | 90 secs

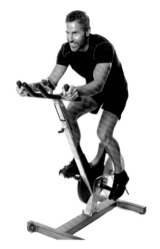

Box Jump

1 | 2 mins
2 | 90 secs

→ Place a 15-25cm raised box on the floor approximately 10-12cm in front of your feet on a non-slip surface. Stand with feet hip-width apart or closer and arms by your sides. Shift your hips backwards then slowly move downwards by hingeing at the knees. Continue to lower yourself until you feel your heels are about to lift up. Keep your head facing the box and position your arms out in front of you for balance. Explode upwards by swinging your arms backward and jumping on to the top of the raised box. Try to keep your feet level with each other and parallel with the floor. Land softly on your mid-foot. Avoid locking your knees on landing.

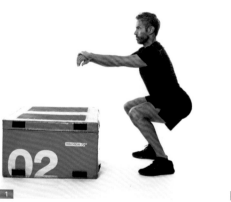

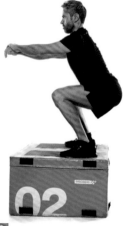

→ Working with a Partner

Working with a partner has many benefits.
In my gyms, I always try to encourage people to
work together in pairs or small support groups

One of the main advantages of having a training partner is the mental benefit that comes from feeling supported. When you have a training partner, your workout goals are no longer simply your own; they are shared goals. The benefit of having shared goals is that emotionally you can rely on each other, and when you are having a bad day your partner is there to help and encourage you through it, and the same applies in return. Having a partner also means you have someone to remind you of good habits and push you that little bit harder each time you work out. The other significant benefit of having a training partner is that there is someone there to check your technique, give you feedback and make sure that you can't hurt yourself. In my gyms, I encourage training partners to video each other doing the big exercises like deadlifts and squats. When you can visualise a move, you can understand how to move better and perform exercises with more control.

Spotting is also a vital role that a training partner can play. Having a spotter on the days when you decide to focus on moving heavy weights can give you the confidence to go for big moves, knowing that someone is there to help you if you can't manage it, or if you become fatigued.

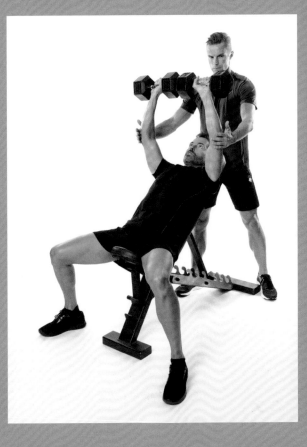

→ Benefits of partner work

The Department of Kinesiology at Indiana University surveyed peope who joined health clubs together and found that people who worked out separately had a 43 per cent dropout rate over the course of a year. Those who worked out together had only a 6.3 per cent drop out rate.

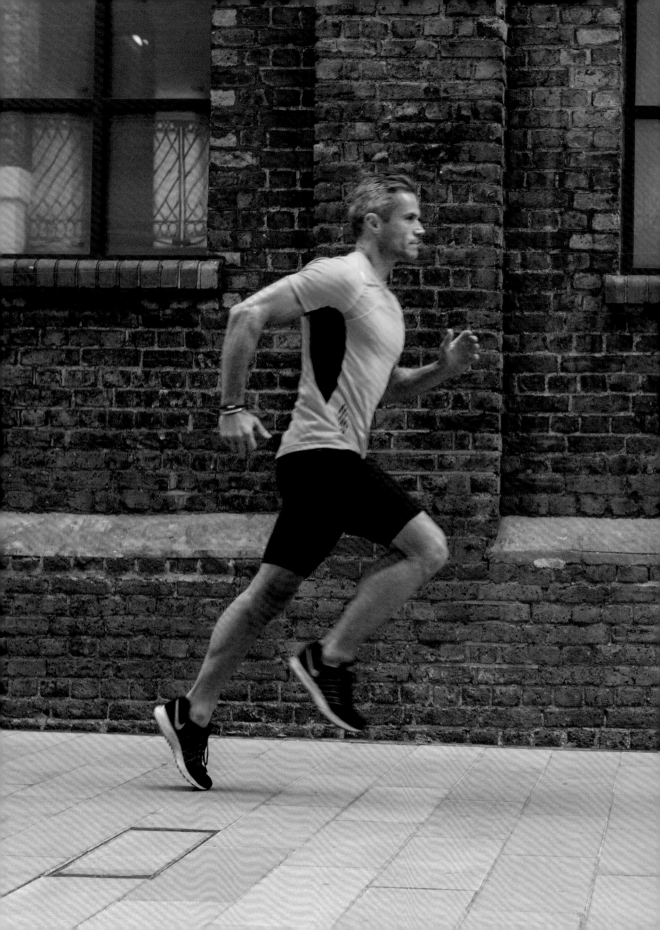

The 8-week Training Programme

Now that you have an idea of the kind of exercises that form the basis of my plan, I am going to outline how they fit into the 8-week programme. On the pages that follow, you will find a page-a-day plan with everything you need – from food to exercise – neatly displayed in a digestible format.

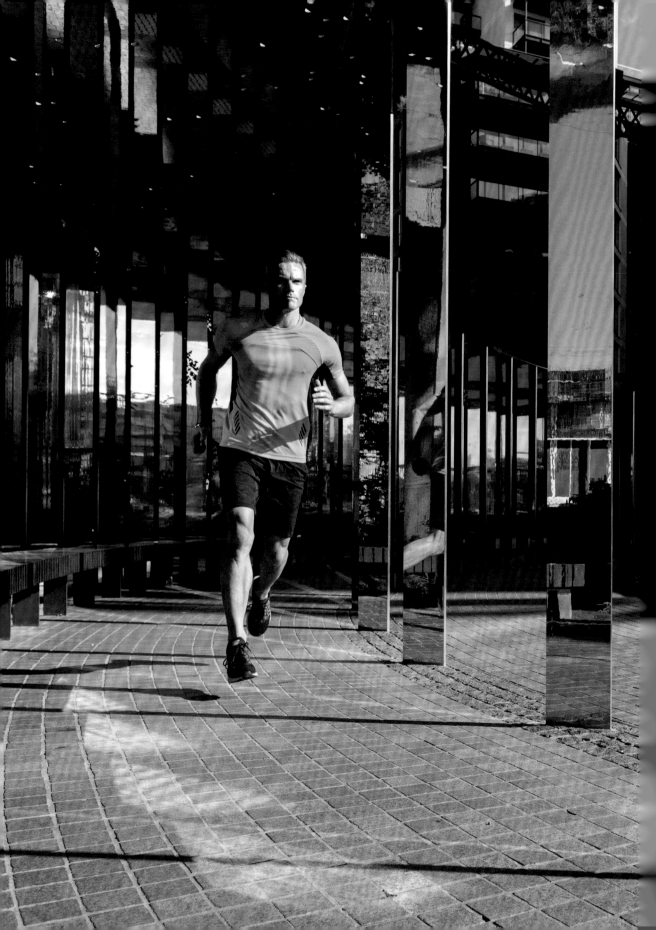

Phase One

In this phase we will prepare the body for the increasingly harder work ahead.

The structure of Phase One will set the format for the 8-week plan. On some days, you will use big, compound strength movements followed by supersets of exercises, and on other days perform strength circuits. Some workout days will end with a metabolic finisher, while on others you will concentrate on strength. For more details, refer to page 27.

In Phase One the rep ranges are high (10-12 reps) in order to maximise muscle and nerve development. More practice allows you to concentrate on the technique of the movements, before starting to load up and move more weight, controlling the stress you put on your body.

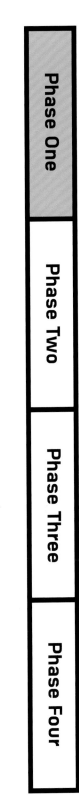

Phase One

Phase Two

Phase Three

Phase Four

Day 01

Today is the first day of your 8-week journey, and you're starting with a strength plus metabolic finisher day (see page 27). Start with the strength focus exercies, performing 10 reps of Trap Bar Deadlift before moving onto Mountain Climber for 30 reps. Alternate for a further four sets before moving onto superset 1, and following the same pattern.

➡ Mobility and activation drills (see pages 100–103)

➡ Main workout

**Strength focus:
5 sets**

1. Trap Bar Deadlift
No. of reps: 10
Tempo: 2:0:2:0
Rest: None

2. Mountain Climber
No. of reps: 30
Tempo: 1:0:2:0
Rest: 90 secs

**Superset 1:
3 sets**

1. Dumbbell Chest Press
No. of reps: 10
Tempo: 2:0:2:0
Rest: None

2. Lat Pull Down
No. of reps: 10
Tempo: 1:0:2:0
Rest: 60 secs

**Superset 2:
3 sets**

1. Weighted Split Squat
No. of reps: 10
Tempo: 2:0:2:0
Rest: None

2. Kettlebell Single Leg Deadlift
No. of reps: 10
Tempo: 2:0:2:0
Rest: 60 secs

**Superset 3:
3 sets**

1. Press-up
No. of reps: to failure
Tempo: 1:0:1:0
Rest: None

2. Single Arm Row
No. of reps: 10
Tempo: 2:0:2:0
Rest: 60 secs

➡ Choose a finisher routine (1, 2 or 3)

Diet Plan

Breakfast:
warm lemon water; 3-egg omelette with 150g spinach and 100g mushrooms; small glass of grapefruit juice

Snack 1:
4 rice cakes and 100g of hummus

Lunch:
150g crab meat with 200g cooked brown rice, palm-sized amount of broccoli, sweet potato and 50g feta cheese

 Vegetarian option: 300g mixed salad with 150g tofu and 70g feta cheese; cup of green tea

Snack 2:
protein smoothie (20g whey, a handful of spinach, 1 pear, 1-2 sticks of celery and a few florets of broccoli)

Dinner:
150g steak (dry cooked in non-stick pan) with 120g broad beans, 120g cabbage and 120g kidney beans

 Vegetarian option: 2 Quorn™ burgers with 120g kale, 120g courgette and 120g broccoli

2 tbsp of quark with 2 tsp honey and a few strawberries

Day
02

As this is your first day of fasting, I would like you to be mindful of how you feel and when your moments of weakness occur. It will help you to plan ahead for future fasting days. It may be that there are tweaks to be made to the hours within which you've scheduled your eating window.

Fasting Diet Plan

Meal 1:
porridge made with 2 tbsp oats with a handful of berries

Meal 2:
150g protein (lean meat, eggs, fish, tofu); mixed salad containing 80g lettuce, 100g kale or spinach and 100g of 2 other raw vegetables, chopped or grated

Meal 3:
150g protein (lean meat, eggs, fish or tofu); mixed salad containing lettuce, 100g kale or spinach and 100g of two other raw vegetables, chopped or grated

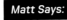

Matt Says:

Don't be afraid of fasting – it's easier than it sounds

Day 03

You may well be feeling a little sore after your first session. This is normal. Delayed onset muscle soreness (or DOMS) tends to strike 48-72 hours after you have worked hard.

Work as hard as you can today as tomorrow you have a day to recover fully.

➡ Mobility and activation drills (see pages 100–103)

➡ Main workout

Strength focus: 5 sets

1. Bench Press
No. of reps: 10
Tempo: 2:0:2:0
Rest: 90 secs

Superset 1: 3 sets

1. Lateral Lunge
No. of reps: 10
Tempo: 1:0:1:0
Rest: None

2. Single Leg Deadlift
No. of reps: 10
Tempo: 1:0:2:0
Rest: 60 secs

Superset 2: 3 sets

1. Seated Cable Row
No. of reps: 10
Tempo: 1:0:2:0
Rest: None

2. Incline Dumbbell Press
No. of reps: 10
Tempo: 1:0:2:0
Rest: 60 secs

Superset 3: 3 sets

1. Reverse Fly
No. of reps: 10
Tempo: 1:0:1:0
Rest: None

2. Triceps Push Down
No. of reps: 10
Tempo: 1:0:1:0
Rest: 60 secs

Diet Plan

Breakfast:
warm lemon water; 150g Greek yoghurt with 1 tsp cashew nut butter and 15 blueberries

Snack 1:
handful of almonds and raisins

Lunch:
150g chicken with 50g edamame beans and 1 tbsp crushed peanuts, 100g quinoa and 100g cooked brown rice

 Vegetarian option: 300g mixed salad with 150g tofu, hemp and flaxseeds, 15 pistachios and 3 tbsp chickpeas

Snack 2:
2 rye crispbreads with cashew nut butter

Dinner:
150g chicken or turkey with 120g spinach, 120g peppers and 100g cooked brown rice

 Vegetarian option: 10 Quorn™ meatballs with 100g cauliflower, 100g purple sprouting broccoli and 100g cooked brown rice

150g probiotic yoghurt with 20 blueberries and 2 tbsp mixed seeds

Day 04

Today is a rest day. Think about keeping a training journal e.g. weights used, reps completed, sets, rest and tempo. In order to progress you need to be aware of where you're progressing from.

Diet Plan

Breakfast:
3 scrambled eggs with ½ an avocado and pinch of zaatar

Snack 1:
apple with 3 tsp almond butter

Lunch:
100g mussels with 100g new potatoes and a rocket salad

 Vegetarian option: bowl of beetroot soup with 1 tbsp Greek yoghurt; protein shake (40g protein powder, 50g spinach and 1 tbsp almond butter)

Snack 2:
unlimited crudités (carrots, cauliflower and broccoli) and 2 tbsp beetroot hummus

Dinner:
150g baked, steamed or poached salmon or trout with 120g kale and 120g celeriac

(V) *Vegetarian option:* green Thai curry with 180g seitan and 120g Tenderstem® broccoli

25g dark chocolate

Matt Says:

Remember that rest is extremely important and needs to be taken seriously

Day 05

Back to the hard work today. You will have noticed that the exercises you are doing vary from day to day – that's the best way to challenge your muscles and keep you mentally and physically on your toes. If you struggle with a new exercise, make sure you master the technique before attempting the full tally of reps and sets.

➡ Mobility and activation drills (see pages 100–103)

➡ Main workout

Strength focus:

1. Pull-up
(banded alternative)
No. of reps: 10
Sets: 5 moving to 6
Tempo: 2:0:2:0
Rest: 90 secs

**Superset 2:
3 sets**

**1. Kettlebell Rack-
Position Squat**
No. of reps: 10
Tempo: 2:0:1:0
Rest: None

**2. Double Kettlebell
Straight Leg
Deadlift**
No. of reps: 10
Tempo: 2:0:1:0
Rest: 60 secs

**Superset 3:
3 sets**

1. Bent Over Row
No. of reps: 10
Tempo: 1:0:2:0
Rest: None

2. Bench Press
No. of reps: 10
Tempo: 1:0:2:0
Rest: 60 secs

**Superset 4:
3 sets**

1. Shoulder Press
No. of reps: 10
Tempo: 1:0:2:0
Rest: None

2. Bicep Curl
No. of reps: 10
Tempo: 1:0:2:0
Rest: 60 secs

➡ Choose a finisher routine (1, 2 or 3)

Diet Plan

Breakfast:
warm lemon water; 2 boiled eggs with 2 pieces of rye toast

Snack 1:
post-workout shake (40g whey, 150ml skimmed milk, ¼ banana, 2 tbsp oats and 2 tsp almond butter)

Lunch:
100g fresh or canned tuna with 6-8 black olives, a handful of spinach, 100g wild rice and 1 beetroot

 Vegetarian option: 100g broccoli, 100g spinach, 100g watercress, 1-2 tomatoes, a sprinkle of hemp seeds, ¼ cucumber and 50g feta cheese

Snack 2:
3 tbsp hummus with 4 sticks celery

Dinner:
150g veal, venison, duck or ostrich (dry cooked in non-stick pan) with 120g broccoli, 1 medium-sized sweet potato and 50-70g chickpeas

Day 06

For today's fast, try to vary the vegetables you have. I ask my clients to introduce a new fruit or vegetable every week. It's a challenge that means they not only get to indulge in new flavours but open up a whole new world of nutrient sources.

Fasting Diet Plan

Meal 1:
porridge made with 2 tbsp oats with a handful of berries

Meal 2:
150g protein (lean meat, fish, eggs or tofu); mixed salad containing lettuce, 100g kale or spinach and 100g of 2 other raw vegetables, chopped or grated

Meal 3:
150g protein (lean meat, eggs, fish or tofu); mixed salad containing 80g lettuce, 100g kale or spinach and 100g of two other raw vegetables, chopped or grated

Day 07

Welcome to your first strength circuits day. As a reminder, you perform the whole of group 1 for the stated number of sets before moving on to group 2. Congratulations are due today – you have almost completed the first week of your 8-week programme. In many ways these will have been the most challenging days of your new regimen.

▣ Mobility and activation drills (see pages 100–103)

▣ Main workout

Group 1: 3 sets

1. Lateral Lunge with Heel Touch
No. of reps: 10
Tempo: explosive
Rest: 30 secs

2. Alternating Spiderman
No. of reps: 30
Tempo: explosive
Rest: 30 secs

3. Burpee
No. of reps: 5
Tempo: explosive
Rest: 30 secs

4. Walking Lunge
No. of reps: 15 (forwards)
Tempo: controlled
Rest: 30 secs

5. Raised Plank with Shoulder Touch
No. of reps: 20-30
Tempo: controlled
Rest: 30 secs

6. Walking Lunge
No. of reps: 15 (backwards)
Tempo: controlled
Rest: 30 secs

7. Raised Plank with Forward Reach
No. of reps: 20-30
Tempo: controlled
Rest: 30 secs

Group 2: 3 sets

1. Box Jump (see page 128)
No. of reps: 15
Tempo: explosive
Rest: 30 secs

2. Single Leg Glute Bridge
No. of reps: 15 (each leg)
Tempo: controlled
Rest: 30 secs

3. Raised Press-up
No. of reps: to failure
Tempo: controlled
Rest: 30 secs

4. Squat Thrust
No. of reps: 10-20
Tempo: explosive
Rest: 30 secs

Diet Plan

Breakfast:
warm lemon water; porridge made with 2 tbsp oats with a handful of raspberries and a handful of blueberries

Snack 1:
protein smoothie (20g protein powder, 150ml semi-skimmed milk, ½ banana, 2 tbsp oats and 2 tsp almond butter)

Lunch:
150g cottage cheese with avocado, pearl barley, raw, thinly sliced red cabbage, chopped kale and kidney beans

Snack 2:
handful of almonds and raisins

Dinner:
chilli with 150g beef or Quorn™ mince, 120g brown rice, 80g kidney beans and spring greens; 25g dark chocolate

Day 08

A rest day today, but make sure you stay active. Studies commissioned by the American Council on Exercise (ACE) and carried out at Western State Colorado University, USA, have shown that active recovery – in which you perform gentle aerobic exercise – helps muscles to bounce back much more quickly. In one trial, participants who jogged to recover from a hard workout found their subsequent performance dropped by only 4.1 per cent compared to 11.8 per cent when they just sat down and did nothing. Aim to walk, go for a gentle jog or cycle or a swim today.

Matt Says:

A gentle walk outside has been shown to raise the spirits and improve your mood

Diet Plan

Breakfast:
4 tbsp nut granola with 100g fat-free Greek yoghurt, 20g protein powder, 15 blueberries and 10 raspberries

Snack 1:
cup of green tea

Lunch:
salad made with 40g goat's cheese, 10 walnuts, 10 olives, 10 cherry tomatoes and 40g beetroot

Snack 2:
60g protein bar

Dinner:
stir-fry with 200g vegetables, 100g chicken or tofu and a handful of peanuts; 150g low-fat Greek yoghurt with raspberries

Day 09

Now nine days into the programme, your body and mind will be beginning to adapt to your new routines. Even if you feel tired before exercising, you may find that your muscles feel less fatigued once you get going. As your circulatory system pumps blood around the body and you become more mobile, you forget how you felt before you started.

➡ Mobility and activation drills (see pages 100–103)

➡ Main workout

Strength focus*:

1. Trap Bar Deadlift
No. of reps: 10
Sets: 6
Tempo: 2:0:2:0
Rest: None

2. Mountain Climber
No. of reps: 30
Sets: 5
Tempo: 1:0:2:0
Rest: 90 secs

Superset 1:
3 sets

1. Dumbbell Chest Press
No. of reps: 10
Tempo: 2:0:2:0
Rest: None

2. Lat Pull Down
No. of reps: 10
Tempo: 1:0:2:0
Rest: 60 secs

Superset 2:
3 sets

1. Weighted Split Squat
No. of reps: 10
Tempo: 2:0:2:0
Rest: None

2. Kettlebell Single Leg Deadlift
No. of reps: 10
Tempo: 2:0:2:0
Rest: 60 secs

Superset 3:
3 sets

1. Press-up
No. of reps: to failure
Tempo: 1:0:1:0
Rest: None

2. Single Arm Row
No. of reps: 10
Tempo: 2:0:2:0
Rest: 60 secs

➡ Choose a finisher routine (1, 2 or 3)

Diet Plan

Breakfast:
warm lemon water; frittata made with 3 eggs, 1 tomato, 50-75g mushrooms, a handful of spinach and 20g cheddar cheese

Snack 1:
100g low-fat Greek yoghurt, 20g whey powder, 30g mixed berries

Lunch:
100g nut roast with 100g parsnips and 120g broccoli

Snack 2:
4 rice cakes and 2 tbsp hummus

Dinner:
150g steak (dry cooked in non stick pan) or non-meat alternative with 100g cabbage, 100g broad beans and 10 new potatoes; 2 kiwi fruits

*Today, you'll alternate your strength focus sets between two exercises, performing six sets of Trap Bar Deadlift and five of Mountain Climber. So you'll finish on Trap Bar Deadlift.

Day
10

You may want to try doing some gentle stretches today. Stretching your major muscle groups – the thighs, hamstrings, calves, chest and back – can leave you feeling invigorated and really help with recovery.

Fasting Diet Plan

Meal 1:
porridge made with 2 tbsp oats and a handful of berries

Meal 2:
150g protein (lean meat, fish or tofu); mixed salad containing 80g lettuce, 100g kale or spinach and 100g of 2 other raw vegetables, chopped or grated

Meal 3:
150g protein (lean meat, fish or tofu); mixed salad containing 80g lettuce, 100g kale or spinach and 100g of 2 other raw vegetables, chopped or grated

Day 11

Back to the hard work. Try to focus on postural control during today's workout. Remember to think about your core abdominal muscles and your coordination as well as your technique. Accidents – and injuries – happen when form is less than adequate so it really matters.

➡ Mobility and activation drills (see pages 100–103)

➡ Main workout

Strength focus:

1. Bench Press
No. of reps: 10
Sets: 5
Tempo: 2:0:2:0
Rest: 90 secs

**Superset 1:
3 sets**

1. Lateral Lunge
No. of reps: 10
Tempo: 1:0:1:0
Rest: None

2. Single Leg Deadlift
No. of reps: 10
Tempo: 1:0:2:0
Rest: 60 secs

**Superset 2:
3 sets**

1. Seated Cable Row
No. of reps: 10
Tempo: 1:0:2:0
Rest: None

2. Incline Dumbbell Press
No. of reps: 10
Tempo: 1:0:2:0
Rest: 60 secs

**Superset 3:
3 sets**

1. Reverse Fly
No. of reps: 10
Tempo: 1:0:1:0
Rest: None

2. Triceps Push Down
No. of reps: 10
Tempo: 1:0:1:0
Rest: 60 secs

Diet Plan

Breakfast:
warm lemon water; Mexican eggs (huevos rancheros) made with 3 eggs, 1 chopped small onion, 1 pepper, 2 tbsp cannellini beans, 1-2 tbsp chopped tomatoes and Tabasco®.

Snack 1:
unlimited vegetable crudités (carrots, cauliflower and broccoli) and 2 tbsp beetroot hummus

Lunch:
150g sliced turkey or tofu with 50g butter beans, 1 small red onion, 1-2 tomatoes, 4 new potatoes; dressing (olive oil, tarragon and basil)

Snack 2:
apple with 3 tsp almond butter

Dinner:
tofu and vegetable patties made with 100g tofu and 100g spinach; 1 medium sweet potato and some celeriac; 2 tbsp quark with 2 tsp honey and a few strawberries

Day 12

Always remember to drink plenty of fluids. My top tip is to buy yourself a water bottle that holds 500ml of fluid and to refill it four times a day. That way you will know you are drinking enough.

Fasting Diet Plan

Meal 1:
porridge made with 2 tbsp oats and a handful of berries

Meal 2:
150g protein (lean meat, fish or tofu); mixed salad containing 80g lettuce, 100g kale or spinach and 100g of two other raw vegetables, chopped or grated

Meal 3:
150g protein (lean meat, fish or tofu); mixed salad containing lettuce, 100g kale or spinach and 100g of two other raw vegetables, chopped or grated

Day 13

You are nearing the end of the first two weeks of your programme. You should be starting to see some noticeable changes both in your appearance and the way you feel. Many of my clients are amazed that, despite the physical challenges, they feel more energised. Not everyone feels that way this quickly, so don't panic if you feel tired. Your time will come.

➡ Mobility and activation drills (see pages 100–103)

➡ Main workout

**Strength focus:
6 sets**

1. Pull-up
No. of reps: 10
Tempo: 2:0:2:0
Rest: 90 secs

**Superset 1:
3 sets**

1. Kettlebell Rack-position Squat
No. of reps: 10
Tempo: 2:0:1:0
Rest: None

2. Double Kettlebell Straight Leg Deadlift
No. of reps: 10
Tempo: 2:0:1:0
Rest: 60 secs

**Superset 2:
3 sets**

1. Bent Over Row
No. of reps: 10
Tempo: 1:0:2:0
Rest: None

2. Bench Press
No. of reps: 10
Tempo: 1:0:2:0
Rest: 60 secs

**Superset 3:
3 sets**

1. Shoulder Press
No. of reps: 10
Tempo: 1:0:2:0
Rest: None

2. Bicep Curl
No. of reps: 10
Tempo: 1:0:2:0
Rest: 60 secs

➡ Choose a finisher routine (1, 2 or 3)

Diet Plan

Breakfast:
warm lemon water; 3-egg omelette with 150g spinach and 100g mushrooms; small glass of grapefruit juice

Snack 1:
4 rice cakes and 2 tbsp hummus

Lunch:
150g roast chicken with 50g edamame beans, 1 tbsp crushed peanuts and 100g quinoa

 Vegetarian option: 300g mixed salad with 150g tofu, hemp and flaxseeds, 15 pistachios and 3 tbsp chickpeas

Snack 2:
2 rye crispbreads with cashew nut butter

Dinner:
10 Quorn™ meatballs with 100g cauliflower, 100g purple sprouting broccoli and 100g brown rice; 150g probiotic yoghurt with 20 blueberries and 2 tbsp mixed seeds

Day 14

Give yourself a pat on the back for reaching the two-week mark. Look back in your training diary and see how far have you come in such a short time.

Matt Says:

It's hugely inspiring to think back to where you started. Progress is the biggest motivator

Diet Plan

Breakfast:
4 tbsp nut granola with 100g fat-free Greek yoghurt, 15 blueberries and 10 raspberries

Snack 1:
4 rice cakes and 2 tbsp beetroot hummus

Lunch:
mussels with 100g new potatoes and a rocket salad

 Vegetarian option: bowl of beetroot soup with 1 tbsp Greek yoghurt; protein shake (40g protein powder, 50g spinach and 1 tbsp almond butter)

Snack 2:
cup of green tea

Dinner:
150g baked, steamed or poached salmon or trout with 120g kale and 120g celeriac

 Vegetarian option: green Thai curry with 180g seitan and 120g Tenderstem® broccoli

2 kiwi fruits

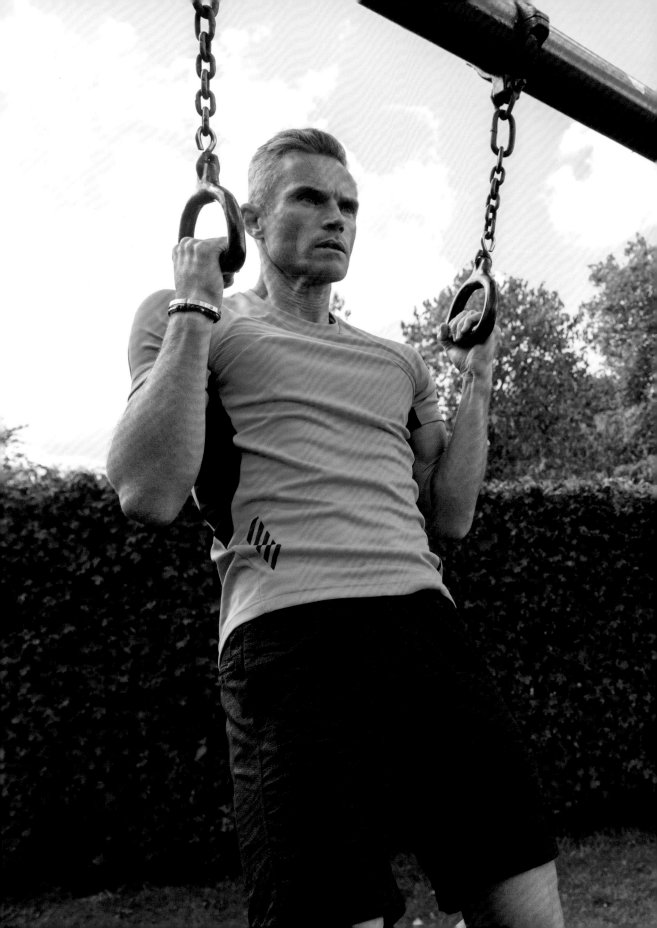

Phase Two

We now start to intensify the strength work and for that initial big compound move I have now lowered the rep range, which means the weight that you move needs to increase. We are now looking to create fatigue after five or six reps, rather than 10 or 12. In Phase Two you need good control. This is a good time to ask a friend or someone who works at your local gym to have a look at your technique.

In the supersets part of the workout, some of the exercises have changed and become more complex. By now you should be moving heavier weights to achieve the fatigue at the required rep ranges.

In the metabolic workouts your recovery time shortens and, when an exercise duration is indicated, you should also be performing more reps of each exercise in the time allowed.

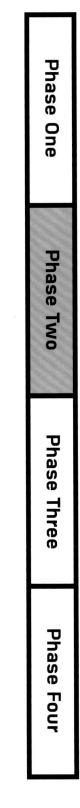

Phase One

Phase Two

Phase Three

Phase Four

Day 15

In this phase we start to move the number of reps down as the weight increases. However, we need to maximise each rep and if the weight is too heavy, you should reduce it.

Pushing yourself is one thing, but pushing yourself beyond your current capabilities is a recipe for disaster. Be patient.

➡ Mobility and activation drills (see pages 100–103)

➡ Main workout

Group 1: 3 sets

1. Lateral Lunge with Heel Touch
No. of reps: 10
Tempo: explosive
Rest: 30 secs

2. Alternating Spiderman
No. of reps: 30
Tempo: explosive
Rest: 30 secs

3. Burpee
No. of reps: 5
Tempo: explosive
Rest: 30 secs

4. Walking Lunge
No. of reps: 15 (forwards)
Tempo: controlled
Rest: 30 secs

5. Raised Plank with Shoulder Touch
No. of reps: 20-30
Tempo: controlled
Rest: 30 secs

6. Walking Lunge
No. of reps: 15 (backwards)
Tempo: controlled
Rest: 30 secs

7. Raised Plank with Forward Reach
No. of reps: 20-30
Tempo: explosive
Rest: 30 secs

Group 2: 3 sets

1. Box Jump (see page 128)
No. of reps: 15
Tempo: explosive
Rest: 30 secs

2. Single Leg Glute Bridge
No. of reps: 15 (each leg)
Tempo: controlled
Rest: 30 secs

3. Raised Press-up
No. of reps: to failure
Tempo: controlled
Rest: 30 secs

4. Squat Thrust
No. of reps: 10-20
Tempo: explosive
Rest: 30 secs

Diet Plan

Breakfast:
warm lemon water; 150g Greek yoghurt with 1 tsp cashew nut butter and 15 blueberries

Snack 1:
a handful of almonds and raisins

Lunch:
150g chicken with 50g edamame beans and 1 tbsp crushed peanuts, 100g quinoa and 100g brown rice,

 Vegetarian option: 300g mixed salad with 150g tofu, hemp and flaxseeds, 15 pistachios and 3 tbsp chickpeas

Snack 2:
protein shake (20g whey, 150ml skimmed milk, 50g spinach and 2 tsp almond butter)

Dinner:
150g veal, venison, duck or ostrich (dry cooked in non-stick pan) with 120g broccoli, 1 medium sweet potato and 50-70g chickpeas

 Vegetarian option: 100g cauliflower egg-fried rice with 120g broccoli and 120g kale.

25g dark chocolate

Day 16

For many people, the dietary aspect of the programme is the hardest to crack. It's not easy and the fasting days, in particular, present a mental challenge. Boredom is one of the main reasons people fail to see a fasting day through, so distract yourself by reading a book or watching a film when you feel hunger pangs coming on.

Matt Says:

Sudoku puzzles, crosswords and books are a great way to unwind and distract yourself when fasting

Fasting Diet Plan

Meal 1:
porridge made with 2 tbsp oats with a handful of berries

Meal 2:
150g protein (lean meat, fish or tofu); mixed salad containing 80g lettuce, 100g kale or spinach and 100g of two other raw vegetables, chopped or grated

Meal 3:
150g protein (lean meat, fish or tofu); mixed salad containing 80g lettuce, 100g kale or spinach and 100g of two other raw vegetables, chopped or grated

Day 17

In this phase of strength building, I want you to aim to lift more weight or achieve another rep each time you come to a workout. I really want you to keep achieving that progressive overload so that the body has to keep developing and giving you the improvemnts you are looking for.

➡ Mobility and activation drills (see pages 100–103)

➡ Main workout

Strength focus:

1. Trap Bar Deadlift
No. of reps: 6
Sets: 6
Tempo: 2:0:2:0
Rest: None

2. Mountain Climber
No. of reps: 30
Sets: 5
Tempo: 1:0:1:0
Rest: 90 secs

**Superset 1:
4 sets**

1. Dumbbell Chest Press
No. of reps: 10
Tempo: 1:0:2:0
Rest: 60 secs

2. Lat Pulldown
No. of reps: 10
Tempo: 2:0:2:0
Rest: 60 secs

**Superset 2:
4 sets**

1. Weighted Split Squat
No. of reps: 10
Tempo: 2:0:2:0
Rest: None

2. Kettlebell Single Leg Deadlift
No. of reps: 10
Tempo: 2:0:2:0
Rest: 60 secs

**Superset 3:
3 sets**

1. Press-up
No. of reps: to failure
Tempo: 1:0:1:0
Rest: None

2. Single Arm Row
No. of reps: 10
Tempo: 2:0:2:0
Rest: 60 secs

➡ Choose a finisher routine (1, 2 or 3)

Diet Plan

Breakfast:
warm lemon water; porridge made with 2 tbsp oats with a handful of raspberries and a handful of blueberries

Snack 1:
a handful of almonds and raisins

Lunch:
300g mixed salad with 150g tofu, hemp and flaxseeds, 15 pistachios and 3 tbsp chickpeas

Snack 2:
2 tbsp red pepper dip with celery

Dinner:
150g non-meat steak, burger or meatball with 100g cabbage, 100g broad beans and 10 new potatoes; 2 tbsp quark with 2 tsp honey and a few raspberries

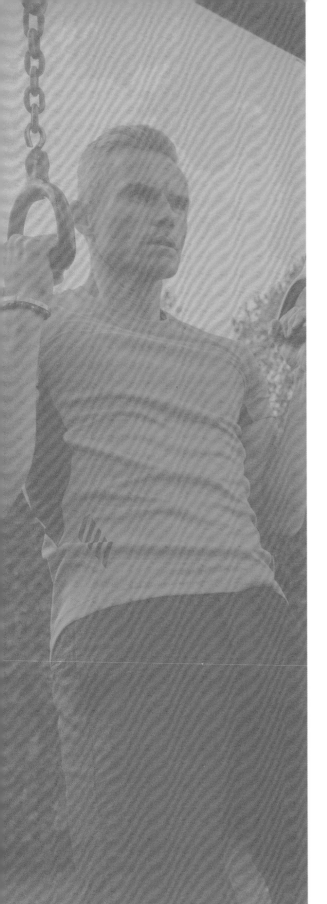

Day
18

If your motivation to fast is flagging, consider this: a 2018 study [1] observed the effects of the same 16:8 fasting ratio we use on this programme on overweight or obese participants for 12 weeks. Participants were allowed to eat any type and quantity of food between the hours of 10am and 6pm, but for the remaining 16 hours they could only drink water or calorie-free beverages. Compared to a different type of fasting, the participants consumed about 350 fewer calories, lost about 3 per cent of their body weight and saw their systolic blood pressure (the standard measure of blood pressure) decrease by about 7 millimeters of mercury (mm Hg). In other words – it works.

Fasting Diet Plan

Meal 1:
porridge made with 2 tbsp oats with a handful of berries

Meal 2:
150g protein (lean meat, fish or tofu); mixed salad containing 80g lettuce, 100g kale or spinach and 100g of two other raw vegetables, chopped or grated

Meal 3:
150g protein (lean meat, fish or tofu); mixed salad containing 80g lettuce, 100g kale or spinach and 100g of two other raw vegetables, chopped or grated

Day 19

Today, watercress is included in your diet plan. This dark green leaf is among my favourite salad ingredients as it not only tastes peppery making it a great flavoursome addition to any salad, but it is rich in antioxidants that can alleviate the natural stress put on our body by a workout. In one eight-week study, a group of healthy subjects were given 85g of watercress – a small bag – and asked to participate in tough exercise. A group consuming no watercress but doing the same workouts acted as a control. Those who had not eaten watercress had more DNA damage than those who had consumed the nutritious green leaf.

➔ Mobility and activation drills (see pages 100–103)

➔ Main workout

**Strength focus:
5 sets**

1. Bench Press
No. of reps: 5
Tempo: 2:0:2:0
Rest: 90 secs
(maximise reps)

**Superset 1:
4 sets**

1. Lateral Lunge
No. of reps: 10
Tempo: 1:1:1:1
Rest: None

2. Single Leg Deadlift
No. of reps: 10
Tempo: 2:0:2:0
Rest: 60 secs

**Superset 2:
4 sets**

1. Seated Cable Row
No. of reps: 10
Tempo: 1:0:2:0
Rest: 60 secs

2. Incline Dumbbell Press
No. of reps: 10
Tempo: 2:0:2:0
Rest: None

**Superset 3:
3 sets**

1. Reverse Fly
No. of reps: 10
Tempo: 1:0:1:0
Rest: None

2. Triceps Push Down
No. of reps: 10
Tempo: 1:0:2:0
Rest: 60 secs

Diet Plan

Breakfast:
warm lemon water; 3-egg omelette with 2 tomatoes, 1 pepper and a handful of spinach

Snack 1:
unlimited vegetable crudités (carrots, cauliflower and broccoli) and 2 tbsp beetroot hummus

Lunch:
100g broccoli, 100g spinach, 100g watercress, 1-2 tomatoes, a sprinkle of hemp seeds, ¼ cucumber and 50g feta cheese

Snack 2:
3 tbsp hummus with 4 sticks of celery

Dinner:
150g veal, venison, duck or ostrich (dry cooked in non-stick pan) with 120g broccoli, 1 medium sweet potato and 50-70g chickpeas

 Vegetarian option: 100g cauliflower egg-fried rice with 120g broccoli and 120g kale

25g dark chocolate

Day
20

Make today a real rest day and don't be tempted to break it with a cardio workout or anything beyond a gentle stroll. Put your feet up and do something you really enjoy.

Diet Plan

Breakfast:
4 tbsp nut granola with 100g low-fat Greek yoghurt, 20g protein powder, 15 blueberries and 10 raspberries

Snack 1:
cup of green tea

Lunch:
salad made with 40g goat's cheese, 10 walnuts, 10 olives, 10 cherry tomatoes and 40g beetroot

Snack 2:
60g protein bar

Dinner:
stir-fry with 200g vegetables, 100g chicken or tofu and a handful of peanuts; 150g low-fat Greek yoghurt with raspberries

Matt Says:

Never feel guilty about sitting back to relax when you are working hard for the rest of the week

Day 21

Today I want you to really focus on being in the present when you are exercising. This is your time to yourself and distractions such as television and iPad screens can add a source of stress to a workout. It is fine to use screens if you find them helpful, but occasionally focus just on the movement and technique you are employing.

➡ Mobility and activation drills (see pages 100–103)

➡ Main workout

**Strength focus:
5 sets**

1. Pull-up
No. of reps: 5 (increase resistance levels)
Tempo: 2:0:2:0
Rest: 90 secs

**Superset 1:
4 sets**

1. Kettlebell Rack-position Squat
No. of reps: 10
Tempo: 2:1:1:1
Rest: None

2. Double Kettlebell Straight Leg Deadlift
No. of reps: 10
Tempo: 2:0:1:0
Rest: 60 secs

**Superset 2:
4 sets**

1. Bent Over Row
No. of reps: 10
Tempo: 1:0:2:0
Rest: None

2. Bench Press
No. of reps: 10
Tempo: 2:0:1:0
Rest: 60 secs

**Superset 3:
4 sets**

1. Shoulder Press
No. of reps: 10
Tempo: 1:0:2:0
Rest: None

2. Bicep Curl
No. of reps: 10
Tempo: 1:0:2:0
Rest: 60 secs

➡ Choose a finisher routine (1, 2 or 3)

Diet Plan

Breakfast:
warm lemon water; Mexican eggs (huevos rancheros) made with 3 eggs, 1 chopped small onion, 1 pepper, 2 tbsp cannellini beans, 1-2 tbsp chopped tomatoes and Tabasco®

Snack 1:
apple with 3 tsp almond butter

Lunch:
150g sliced turkey or vegetarian cheese with 50g butter beans, 1 small red onion, 1-2 tomatoes, 4 cold new potatoes; dressing (olive oil, tarragon and basil)

Snack 2:
300g mixed salad with 3-4 florets broccoli, 1 tsp flaxseeds and 50g ricotta cheese

Dinner:
tofu and vegetable patties made with 100g tofu and 100g spinach; 1 medium sweet potato and some celeriac; 2 tbsp quark with 2 tsp honey and a few strawberries

Day 22

Remind yourself that every small step is a step towards a younger, fitter and stronger you. So resist the temptation to stray away from your daily fast, and take control of your diet. That is the route to success.

Fasting Diet Plan

Meal 1:
porridge made with 2 tbsp oats with a handful of berries

Meal 2:
150g protein (lean meat, fish or tofu); mixed salad containing 80g lettuce, 100g kale or spinach and 100g of two other raw vegetables, chopped or grated

Meal 3:
150g protein (lean meat, fish or tofu); mixed salad containing 80g lettuce, 100g kale or spinach and 100g of two other raw vegetables, chopped or grated

Day 23

Today I want you to think about maintaining good technique as muscles get fatigued. The weights you are lifting are heavy and you have very little recovery time between moves. That is precisely when technique can slip, so be aware.

⊡ Mobility and activation drills (see pages 100–103)

⊡ Main workout

Group 1: 3 sets

1. Lateral Lunge with Heel Touch
No. of reps: 10 each leg
Tempo: explosive
Rest: 30 seconds

2. Alternating Spiderman
No. of reps: 30
Tempo: controlled
Rest: 30 seconds

3. Burpee
No. of reps: 5
Tempo: explosive
Rest: 30 seconds

4. Walking Lunge
No. of reps: 15 steps (forwards)
Tempo: controlled
Rest: 30 seconds

5. Raised Plank with Shoulder Touch
No. of reps: 20-30
Tempo: controlled
Rest: 30 seconds

6. Walking Lunge
No. of reps: 15 steps (backwards)
Tempo: controlled
Rest: 30 seconds

7. Raised Plank with Forward Reach
No. of reps: 20-30
Tempo: controlled
Rest: 30 seconds

Group 2: 3 sets

1. Box Jump (see page 128)
No. of reps: 15
Tempo: explosive
Rest: 30 seconds

2. Single Leg Glute Bridge
No. of reps: 15 each leg
Tempo: controlled
Rest: 30 seconds

3. Raised Press-up
No. of reps: to failure
Tempo: controlled
Rest: 30 seconds

4. Squat Thrust
No. of reps: 10-20
Tempo: explosive
Rest: 30 seconds

Diet Plan

Breakfast:
warm lemon water; 2 boiled eggs with 2 pieces of rye toast

 Vegetarian option: add 10 BCAA capsules

Snack 1:
protein shake with 40g protein powder

Lunch:
100g fresh or canned tuna with 6-8 black olives, a handful of spinach, 100g wild rice and 1 beetroot

 Vegetarian option: 100g broccoli, 100g spinach, 100g watercress, 1-2 tomatoes, a sprinkle of hemp seeds, ¼ cucumber and 50g feta cheese

Snack 2:
3 tbsp hummus with 4 sticks of celery

Dinner:
150g veal, venison, duck or ostrich (dry cooked in non-stick pan) with 120g broccoli, 1 medium sweet potato and 50-70g chickpeas

 Vegetarian option: 100g cauliflower egg-fried rice with 120g broccoli and 120g kale

2 kiwi fruits

Day 24

I am a big fan of beetroot hummus and pretty much anything else containing the earthy deep purple vegetable. Not only is beetroot a good source of iron and folate (naturally occurring folic acid), but it also contains nitrates that researchers have shown can help lower blood pressure, boost exercise performance and recovery, and enhance brain health.

Diet Plan

Breakfast:
4 tbsp nut granola with 100g fat-free Greek yoghurt, 15 blueberries and 10 raspberries

Snack 1:
4 rice cakes and 2-3 tbsp beetroot hummus

Lunch:
100g mussels with 100g new potatoes and a rocket salad

(V) *Vegetarian option:* bowl of beetroot soup with 1 tbsp Greek yoghurt; protein shake (40g protein powder, 50g spinach and 1 tbsp almond butter)

Snack 2:
cup of green tea

Dinner:
150g baked, steamed or poached salmon or trout with 120g kale and 120g celeriac

(V) *Vegetarian option:* green Thai curry with 180g seitan and 120g Tenderstem® broccoli

2 kiwi fruits

Matt Says:

A good breakfast is an essential start to the day and really fires up your metabolism

Day 25

Experiment with making your own protein shakes. In one study conducted at the University of Nottingham [2], muscle building was shown to increase in men when they consumed whey protein after a weights session, regardless of whether the weights they lifted were heavy or light.

◰ Mobility and activation drills (see pages 100–103)

◰ Main workout

Strength focus:

1. Trap Bar Deadlift
No. of reps: 6
Sets: 6
Tempo: 2:0:2:0
Rest: None

2. Mountain Climber
No. of reps: 30
Sets: 5
Tempo: 1:0:1:0
Rest: 90 secs

Superset 1:
4 sets

1. Dumbbell Chest Press
No. of reps: 10
Tempo: 1:0:2:0
Rest: 60 secs

2. Lat Pull Down
No. of reps: 10
Tempo: 2:0:2:0
Rest: 60 secs

Superset 2:
4 sets

1. Weighted Split Squat
No. of reps: 10
Tempo: 2:0:2:0
Rest: None

2. Kettlebell Single Leg Deadlift
No. of reps: 10
Tempo: 2:0:2:0
Rest: 60 secs

Superset 3:
3 sets

1. Press-up
No. of reps: to failure
Tempo: 1:0:1:0
Rest: None

2. Single Arm Row
No. of reps: 10
Tempo: 2:0:2:0
Rest: 60 secs

◰ Choose a finisher routine (1, 2 or 3)

Diet Plan

Breakfast:
warm lemon water; 150g Greek yoghurt with 1 tsp cashew nut butter and 15 raspberries

Snack 1:
post-workout shake (20g of whey, 150ml skimmed milk, ¼ banana, 2 tbsp oats and 2 tsp almond butter)

Lunch:
salad made with 40g goat's cheese, 10 walnuts, 10 olives, 10 cherry tomatoes and 40g beetroot

Dinner:
150g veal, venison, duck or ostrich (dry cooked in non-stick pan) with 120g broccoli, 1 medium sweet potato and 50-70g chickpeas

 Vegetarian option: 100g cauliflower egg-fried rice with 120g broccoli and 120g kale

25g dark chocolate

Day 26

Make blueberries one of the berries you add to your porridge. They are rammed with antioxidants and scientists have shown they may help improve rate of recovery from intense exercise [3]. Studies have also associated blueberries with improved brain health [4] and inhibiting fat cell development [5, 6].

Fasting Diet Plan

Meal 1:
porridge made with 2 tbsp oats with a handful of berries

Meal 2:
150g protein (lean meat, fish or tofu); mixed salad containing 80g lettuce, 100g kale or spinach and 100g of two other raw vegetables, chopped or grated

Meal 3:
150g protein (lean meat, fish or tofu); mixed salad containing 80g lettuce, 100g kale or spinach and 100g of two other raw vegetables, chopped or grated

Matt Says:

Remember, even on a fasting day you are packing in nutrients essential for your health

Day 27

You are almost half-way through the programme and are likely getting used to the exercise regimen. Hopefully you will have begun to adjust to your new daily and weekly routine. Just make sure that you are putting in 100 per cent effort from now on in, not just going through the motions. It's easy to think you are doing 'enough' to make a difference, but let's keep in mind how significant you want that difference to be. Make sure you are being as good as you can be with every single repetition today and for the remaining sessions.

➡ Mobility and activation drills (see pages 100–103)

➡ Main workout

Strength focus: 5 sets

1. Bench Press
No. of reps: 5
Tempo: 2:0:2:0
Rest: 90 secs
(maximise reps)

Superset 1: 4 sets

1. Lateral Lunge
No. of reps: 10
Tempo: 1:1:1:1
Rest: None

2. Single Leg Deadlift
No. of reps: 10
Tempo: 2:0:2:0
Rest: 60 secs

Superset 2: 4 sets

1. Seated Cable Row
No. of reps: 10
Tempo: 1:0:2:0
Rest: 60 secs

2. Incline Dumbbell Press
No. of reps: 10
Tempo: 2:0:2:0
Rest: None

Superset 3: 3 sets

1. Reverse Fly
No. of reps: 10
Tempo: 1:0:1:0
Rest: None

2. Triceps Push Down
No. of reps: 10
Tempo: 1:0:2:0
Rest: 60 secs

Diet Plan

Breakfast:
warm lemon water; 4 tbsp nut granola with 100g fat-free Greek yoghurt and 2 tbsp mixed berries

Snack 1:
4 rice cakes and 2 tbsp beetroot hummus

Lunch:
100g mussels with 100g new potatoes and rocket salad

 Vegetarian option: bowl of beetroot soup with 1 tbsp Greek yoghurt; protein shake (40g protein, 50g spinach and 1 tbsp almond butter)

Snack 2:
cup of green tea

Dinner:
150g baked, steamed or poached salmon or trout with 120g kale and 120g celeriac

 Vegetarian option: green Thai curry with 180g seitan and 120g Tenderstem® broccoli

25g dark chocolate

Day
28

Congratulations – you are half way through your 8-week plan. You are probably feeling and looking better already, but you really can make the programme work for you by focusing on every detail in the remaining four weeks. Keep up the good work.

Fasting Diet Plan

Meal 1:
porridge made with 2 tbsp oats with a handful of berries

Meal 2:
150g protein (lean meat, fish or tofu); mixed salad containing 80g lettuce, 100g kale or spinach and 100g of two other raw vegetables, chopped or grated

Meal 3:
150g protein (lean meat, fish or tofu); mixed salad containing 80g lettuce, 100g kale or spinach and 100g of two other raw vegetables, chopped or grated

Matt Says:

There's no turning back now – you have done the hardest part, so keep going

Day 29

As the weights we use increase, it is essential that we think about how we 'ground' the exercises we do. What I mean by 'grounding' is the contact and control that we have on to and into the floor. We have talked about bracing on page 114, and grounding is part of the same process. Whenever you do any exercise, creating a feeling of bracing or grounding and then engaging the core muslces before you move will allow you to move more weight and feel safer and more in control as you do so.

➡ Mobility and activation drills (see pages 100–103)

➡ Main workout

**Strength focus:
5 sets**

1. Pull-up
No. of reps: 5
(increase resistance
levels; here you
should be using your
full body weight or
even adding to your
body weight)
Tempo: 2:0:2:0
Rest: 90 secs

**Superset 1:
4 sets**

**1. Kettlebell Rack-
position Squat**
No. of reps: 10
Tempo: 2:1:1:1
Rest: None

**2. Double Kettlebell
Straight Leg
Deadlift**
No. of reps: 10
Tempo: 2:0:1:0
Rest: 60 secs

**Superset 2:
4 sets**

1. Bent Over Row
No. of reps: 10
Tempo: 1:0:2:0
Rest: None

2. Bench Press
No. of reps: 10
Tempo: 2:0:1:0
Rest: 60 secs

**Superset 3:
4 sets**

1. Shoulder Press
No. of reps: 10
Tempo: 1:0:2:0
Rest: None

2. Bicep Curl
No. of reps: 10
Tempo: 1:0:2:0
Rest: 60 secs

➡ Choose a finisher routine (1, 2 or 3)

Diet Plan

Breakfast:
warm lemon water; frittata made with 3 eggs,
1 tomato, 50-75g mushrooms, a handful of spinach
and 20g cheddar cheese

Snack 1:
100g fat-free Greek yoghurt, 20g whey powder
and 30g mixed berries

Lunch:
300g mixed salad with 150g tofu, hemp and
flaxseeds, 15 pistachios and 3 tbsp chickpeas

Snack 2:
4 rice cakes and 2 tbsp hummus

Dinner:
150g non-meat steak, burger or meatball with
100g cabbage, 100g broad beans and 10 new
potatoes; 2 kiwi fruits

Day 30

You will have noticed by now that eggs are featuring prominently in my eating plan. That's because they are such a compact powerhouse of nutrients – packed with protein and dozens of important vitamins and minerals. Nutritionists have certainly changed their opinion on eggs in recent years and now studies have confirmed that regular egg-eaters are healthier than the rest of the population. One study [7] showed that people who consume an egg a day could significantly reduce their risk of cardiovascular diseases compared with eating no eggs. All the more reason to make them a mainstay.

Diet Plan

Breakfast:
warm lemon water; 3-egg omelette with 150g spinach and 100g mushrooms; small glass of grapefruit juice

Snack 1:
apple with 3 tsp almond butter

Lunch:
150g chicken with 50g edamame beans, 1 tbsp crushed peanuts and 100g quinoa

Snack 2:
2 rye crispbreads with cashew nut butter

Dinner:
10 Quorn™ meatballs with 100g cauliflower and 100g purple sprouting broccoli; 125g probiotic yoghurt with 20 blueberries and 2 tbsp mixed seeds

Matt Says:

Often, the most nutrient packed foods are the most natural

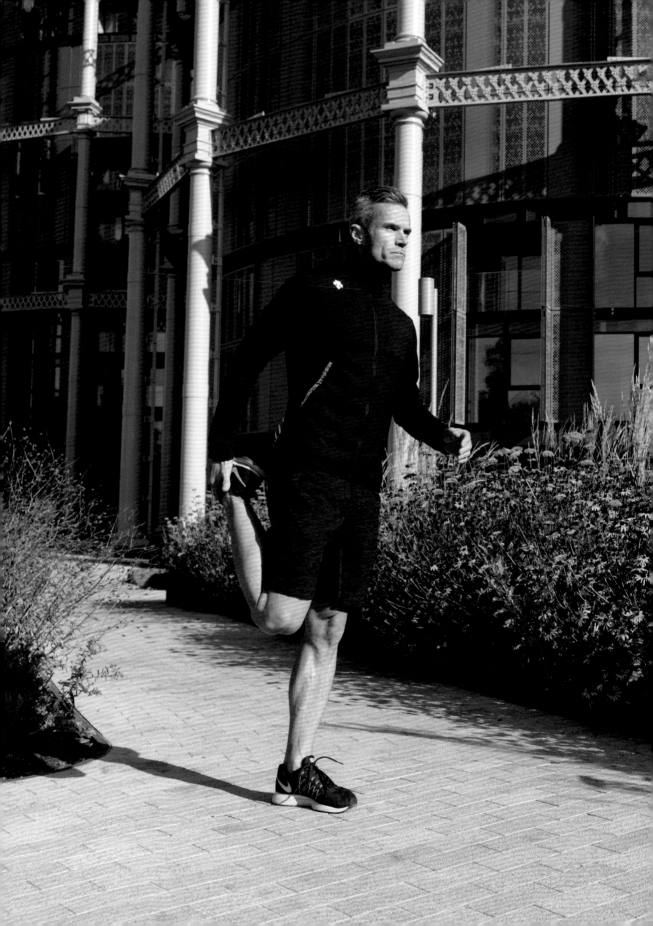

Phase Three

In Phase Three we are looking to push the strength and muscle development that bit further. Two main changes will be an even lower rep range and therefore increased weight, and greater time lifting under tension. You will see that I have increased the amount of time the eccentric phase of the move takes. This extra tension on the muscles really helps to encourage greater muscle adaptation.

Phase One

Phase Two

Phase Three

Phase Four

Day 31

In this phase, make sure to maximise the effort in each rep, reducing weight if necessary. Progressively heavier weights are all part of our goal to increase your hormonal production and boost your metabolism, so stick with them if you can.

▣ Mobility and activation drills (see pages 100–103)

▣ Main workout

Strength focus:

1. Trap Bar Deadlift
No. of reps: 10, warm-up, 6, 5, 4, 3, 4 ,5
Sets: 7
Tempo: 1:0:3:0
Rest: None

2. Mountain Climber
No. of reps: 30
Sets: 5
Tempo: controlled
Rest: 90 secs

Superset 1:
4 sets

1. Bench Press
No. of reps: 10
Tempo: 3:0:1:0
(eccentric slow)
Rest: None

2. Pull-up
No. of reps: to failure
Tempo: controlled
Rest: 60 secs

Superset 2:
4 sets

1. Weighted Split Squat
No. of reps: 10
Tempo: 2:0:2:0
Rest: None

2. Nordic Curl
No. of reps: 10
Tempo: slow eccentric
Rest: 60 secs

Superset 3:
4 sets

1. Press-up
No. of reps: to failure
Tempo: 1:0:1:0
Rest: None

2. Lat Pulldown
No. of reps: 10
Tempo: 2:0:2:0
Rest: 60 secs

▣ Choose a finisher routine (1, 2 or 3)

Diet Plan

Breakfast:
warm lemon water; Mexican eggs (huevos rancheros) made with 3 eggs, 1 chopped small onion, 1 pepper, 2 tbsp cannellini beans, 1-2 tbsp chopped tomatoes and Tabasco®

Snack 1:
100g fat-free Greek yoghurt, 20g whey powder, 30g mixed berries

Lunch:
100g of fresh or canned tuna with 6-8 black olives, a handful of spinach, 80g brown rice and 3-4 florets of broccoli

Snack 2:
4 rice cakes and 2 tbsp hummus

Dinner:
150g steak or non-meat alternative with 100g cabbage, 100g broad beans and 10 new potatoes; 2 kiwi fruits

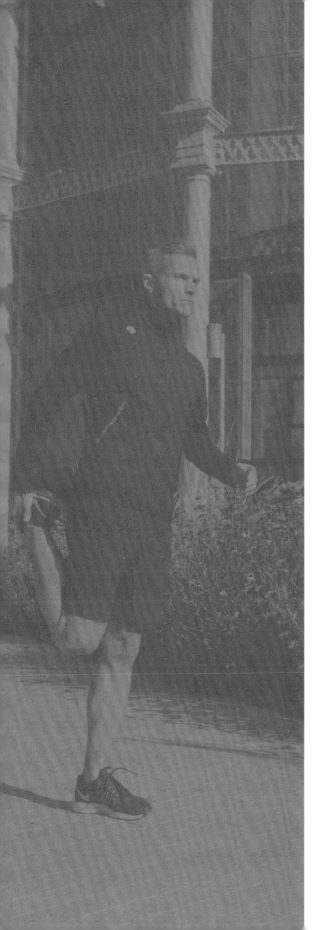

Day
32

To take your mind of fasting today, let's construct a personal audit. Ask yourself: how much water and healthy fluids you are drinking? Are you getting sufficient sleep that you feel fully rested when you wake up? Are you sticking to your meal schedule and managing to avoid additional snacking on workout days? It's always good to review how things are going and to make tweaks where appropriate.

Fasting Diet Plan

Meal 1:
porridge made with 2 tbsp oats with a handful of berries

Meal 2:
150g protein (lean meat, fish or tofu); mixed salad containing 80g lettuce, 100g kale or spinach and 100g of two other raw vegetables, chopped or grated

Meal 3:
150g protein (lean meat, fish or tofu); mixed salad containing 80g lettuce, 100g kale or spinach and 100g of two other raw vegetables, chopped or grated

Matt Says:

Hydration is something many people overlook – make sure you take on fluids

Day 33

At this point in the programme, we want to really focus on pushing your strength levels one stage further. That's why you'll now see that the rep ranges on our strength-focused movements start to reduce. You should also be upping the weight that you are pushing and pulling. You will find that there will be an increased requirement for bracing, and a heavier workload on all of the muscles you are using in each of your movements.

▶ Mobility and activation drills (see pages 100–103)

▶ Main workout

**Strength focus:
6 sets**

1. Bench Press
No. of reps: 10 warm-up, 6, 5, 4, 3, 2
Tempo: 3:0:1:0
(eccentric slow)
Rest: 90 secs

**Superset 1:
4 sets**

1. Lateral Lunge
No. of reps: 10
Tempo: 1:1:1:1
Rest: None

**2. Single Leg
Deadlift**
No. of reps: 10
Tempo: 3:0:1:0
Rest: 60 secs

**Superset 2:
4 sets**

1. Dumbbell Press
No. of reps: 10
Tempo: 3:0:1:0
(eccentric slow)
Rest: None

2. Dumbbell Pullover
No. of reps: 10
Tempo: 3:0:1:0
Rest: 60 secs

**Superset 3:
4 sets**

1. Face Pull
No. of reps: 10
Tempo: 3:0:1:0
(eccentric slow)
Rest: None

2. Triceps Push Down
No. of reps: 10
Tempo: 2:0:3:0
Rest: 60 secs

Diet Plan

Breakfast:
warm lemon water; porridge made with 2 tbsp oats with a handful of berries

Snack 1:
a handful of almonds and raisins

Lunch:
300g mixed salad with 150g prawns or tofu, hemp and flaxseeds, 15 pistachios and 3 tbsp chickpeas

Snack 2:
unlimited vegetable crudités (carrots, cauliflower and broccoli) and 2 tbsp beetroot hummus

Dinner:
150g turkey with 50g celeriac, a handful of fine beans and 10 new potatoes; 2 tbsp quark with 2 tsp honey and a few raspberries

Day
34

All broccoli is good for you, so why do I recommend Tenderstem®? It's because it's been shown to contain the highest levels of beneficial glucosinolates – the potent chemicals understood to have cancer-fighting properties – compared to the ten other Brassica varieties tested in research. If you can't find it, any variety of broccoli is better than none.

Diet Plan

Breakfast:
warm lemon water; 2 boiled eggs with 2 pieces of rye toast

Snack 1:
apple with 3 tsp almond butter

Lunch:
100g mussels with 100g new potatoes and a rocket salad

 Vegetarian option: 100g nut roast with 100g parsnips and 120g broccoli

Snack 2:
4 rice cakes and 2 tbsp hummus

Dinner:
150g baked, steamed or poached salmon or trout with 120g kale and 120g celeriac

 Vegetarian option: green Thai curry with 180g seitan and 120g Tenderstem® broccoli

2 kiwi fruits

Matt Says:

Your snacks can be mix and matched – don't force yourself to eat one you really don't like

Day 35

Three weeks until you complete the programme. Well done for making it this far. You have a day off tomorrow, so make sure you push it hard today and make it worth your time.

▶ Mobility and activation drills (see pages 100–103)

▶ Main workout

Strength focus:

1. Squat
No. of reps: 5
Sets: 5
Tempo: 3:1:1:0
(eccentric slow)
Rest: 90 secs

**Superset 1:
4 sets**

1. Incline Dumbbell Press
No. of reps: 10
Tempo: 1:0:3:0
(eccentric slow)
Rest: None

2. Single Arm Row
No. of reps: 10
Tempo: 1:0:3:0
(eccentric slow)
Rest: 60 secs

**Superset 2:
4 sets**

1. Shoulder Press
No. of reps: 10
Tempo: 1:0:3:0
Rest: None

2. Bicep Curl
No. of reps: 10
Tempo: 1:0:3:0
(eccentric slow)
Rest: None

**Superset 3
4 sets**

1. Shoulder Press
No. of reps: 10
Tempo: 1:0:3:0
Rest: None

2. Hammer Curl
No. of reps: 10
Tempo: 1:0:3:0
Rest: 60 secs

▶ Choose a finisher routine (1, 2 or 3)

Diet Plan

Breakfast:
4 tbsp nut granola with 100g fat-free Greek yoghurt, 20g protein powder, 15 blueberries and 10 raspberries

Snack 1:
2 tbsp beetroot dip with red pepper

Lunch:
salad made with 40g goat's cheese, 10 walnuts, 10 olives, 10 cherry tomatoes and 20g beetroot

Snack 2:
a handful of almonds and raisins

Dinner:
150g steak (dry-cooked in non-stick pan) or non-meat alternative with 1 medium sweet potato, a handful of kale, a handful of celeriac and 75g kidney beans; 2 tbsp quark with 2 tsp honey and a handful of berries

Day 36

If you're struggling at the prospect of another fasting day, let's remind ourselves why we are doing it. Fasting for short periods can hike up the production of male hormones and this effect is enhanced in combination with exercise. One study [8] showed that a day of fasting increased HGH by 2000 per cent in a group of men, and another [9] indicated that it has a remarkable correlation with testosterone levels. Keep it up!

Fasting Diet Plan

Meal 1:
porridge made with 2 tbsp oats with a handful of berries

Meal 2:
150g protein (lean meat, fish or tofu); mixed salad containing 80g lettuce, 100g kale or spinach and 100g of two other raw vegetables, chopped or grated

Meal 3:
150g protein (lean meat, fish or tofu); mixed salad containing 80g lettuce, 100g kale or spinach and 100g of two other raw vegetables, chopped or grated

Day 37

Think about the time of day that you exercise. Is it really the best time for you? Try to fit in workouts at a time when it most suits your mood and other commitments – it means you will get more out of your efforts if you are emotionally ready and prepared.

➔ Mobility and activation drills (see pages 100–103)

➔ Main workout

Group 1: 3 sets

1. Lateral lunge with Heel Touch
No. of reps: 10 each leg
Tempo: explosive
Rest: 30 secs

2. Alternating Spiderman
No. of reps: 30
Tempo: controlled
Rest: 30 secs

3. Burpee
No. of reps: 5
Tempo: explosive
Rest: 30 secs

4. Walking Lunge
No. of reps: 15 steps (forwards)
Tempo: controlled
Rest: 30 secs

5. Raised Plank with Shoulder Touch
No. of reps: 20-30
Tempo: controlled
Rest: 30 secs

6. Walking Lunge
No. of reps: 15 steps (backwards)
Tempo: controlled
Rest: 30 secs

7. Raised Plank with Shoulder Touch
No. of reps: 20-30
Tempo: controlled
Rest: 30 secs

Group 2: 3 sets

1. Box Jump (see page 128)
No. of reps: 15
Tempo: explosive
Rest: 30 secs

2. Single Leg Glute Bridge
No. of reps: 15 each leg
Tempo: controlled
Rest: 30 secs

3. Raised Press-up
No. of reps: to failure
Tempo: controlled
Rest: 30 secs

4. Squat Thrust
No. of reps: 10-20
Tempo: explosive
Rest: 30 secs

Diet Plan

Breakfast:
warm lemon water; porridge made with 2 tbsp oats with a handful each of raspberries and blueberries

Snack 1:
protein smoothie (20g protein powder, 150ml semi-skimmed milk, ½ banana, 2 tbsp oats and 2 tsp almond butter)

Lunch:
100g mussels with 100g new potatoes and a rocket salad

Snack 2:
4 rice cakes and 2 tbsp beetroot hummus

Dinner:
150g salmon with a handful of fine beans, a handful of spinach and 80g brown rice; 2 tbsp plain yoghurt and handful of berries

Day
38

No exercise is scheduled for today, so enjoy the rest. Reward yourself by being outside. Greenery and open spaces are as good for the mind as they are for the body, so enjoy it.

Fasting Diet Plan

Meal 1:
porridge made with 2 tbsp oats with a handful of berries

Meal 2:
150g protein (lean meat, fish or tofu); mixed salad containing 80g lettuce, 100g kale or spinach and 100g of two other raw vegetables, chopped or grated

Meal 3:
150g protein (lean meat, fish or tofu); mixed salad containing 80g lettuce, 100g kale or spinach and 100g of two other raw vegetables, chopped or grated

Matt Says:

It's remarkable how the human body adapts to consuming less food. Fasting will now be getting easier, I am sure

Day 39

An independent study [10] conducted by exercise physiologists at the University of Wisconsin and commissioned by the American Council on Exercise, a not-for-profit consumer watchdog, showed that the Bench Press is among the most effective exercises for targeting the major muscles of the chest. And, of course, that means minimising those moobs. Concentrate fully on getting technique right today to maximise the effects.

▣ Mobility and activation drills (see pages 100–103)

▣ Main workout

Strength focus:

1. Trap Bar Deadlift
No. of reps: 10, 6, 5, 4, 3, 4, 5
Sets: 7
Tempo: 1:0:3:0
Rest: None

2. Mountain Climber
No. of reps: 30
Sets: 5
Tempo: controlled
Rest: 90 secs

Superset 1:
4 sets

1. Bench Press
No. of reps: 10
Tempo: 3:0:1:0 (eccentric slow)
Rest: None

2. Pull-up
No. of reps: to failure
Tempo: controlled
Rest: 60 secs

Superset 2
4 sets

1. Weighted Split Squat
No. of reps: 10
Tempo: 2:0:2:0
Rest: None

2. Nordic Curl
No. of reps: 10
Tempo: slow eccentric
Rest: 60 secs

Superset 3:
4 sets

1. Press-up
No. of reps: to failure
Tempo: 1:0:1:0
Rest: None

2. Lat Pulldown
No. of reps: 10
Tempo: 2:0:2:0
Rest: 60 secs

▣ Choose a finisher routine (1, 2 or 3)

Diet Plan

Breakfast:
warm lemon water; 3 scrambled eggs with ½ an avocado and a sprinkle of zaatar

Snack 1:
4 rice cakes and 2 tbsp hummus

Lunch:
150g chicken with 120g broccoli and 120g cauliflower

 Vegetarian option: 100g nut roast with 100g parsnips and 120g broccoli

Snack 2:
apple with 3 tsp almond butter

Dinner:
150g non-meat steak, burger or meatball with 100g cabbage, 100g broad beans and 10 new potatoes; 2 kiwi fruits

Day 40

Twenty steamed mussels provide 4.7mg of zinc, a mineral essential to help make the enzymes needed for cell division, growth, wound healing and a healthy immune system. Zinc is also crucial for healthy sperm which is why men need an intake of 9.5mg a day of zinc. Mussels also taste incredible, so enjoy the treat on this rest day.

Diet Plan

Breakfast:
warm lemon water; 4 tbsp nut granola with 100g Greek yoghurt, 15 blueberries and 10 raspberries

Snack 1:
4 rice cakes and 2 tbsp beetroot hummus

Lunch:
mussels with 100g new potatoes and a rocket salad

(V) *Vegetarian option:* one bowl beetroot soup with 1 tbsp Greek yoghurt; protein shake (40g protein powder, 50g spinach and 1 tbsp almond butter)

Snack 2:
cup of green tea

Dinner:
150g baked, steamed or poached salmon or trout with 120g kale and 120g celeriac

(V) *Vegetarian option:* green Thai curry with 180g seitan and 120g Tenderstem® broccoli

Matt Says:

Use apps to send alerts to remind you to stand up and move at work

Day 41

I will regularly advise you to sprinkle seeds on your yoghurt or porridge. Why? Well, they are not only a valuable source of protein and healthy fats, but are packed with the minerals we men need to enhance hormone production.

Pumpkin seeds are a favourite of mine as they contain high levels of zinc, low levels of which can cause a drop in testosterone levels in a matter of weeks.

➡ Mobility and activation drills (see pages 100–103)

➡ Main workout

Strength focus: **6 sets**	**Superset 1:** **4 sets**	**Superset 2:** **4 sets**	**Superset 3:** **4 sets**
1. Bench Press No. of reps: 10, 6, 5, 4, 3, 2 Tempo: 3:0:1:0 (eccentric slow) Rest: 90 secs	**1. Lateral Lunge** No. of reps: 10 Tempo: 1:1:1:1 Rest: None **2. Single Leg Deadlift** No. of reps: 10 Tempo: 3:0:1:0 Rest: 60 secs	**1. Dumbbell Chest Press** No. of reps: 10 Tempo: 3:0:1:0 (eccentric slow) Rest: None **2. Dumbbell Pullover** No. of reps: 10 Tempo: 3:0:1:0 Rest: 60 secs	**1. Face Pull** No. of reps: 10 Tempo: 3:0:1:0 (eccentric slow) Rest: None **2. Triceps Push Down** No. of reps: 10 Tempo: 2:0:3:0 Rest: 60 secs

Diet Plan

Breakfast:
warm lemon water; 150g Greek yoghurt with 1 tsp cashew nut butter and 15 blueberries

Snack 1:
a handful of almonds and raisins

Lunch:
150g chicken with 50g edamame beans, 1 tbsp crushed peanuts, 100g quinoa and 100g brown rice

 Vegetarian option: 300g mixed salad with 150g tofu, hemp and flaxseeds, 15 pistachios and 3 tbsp chickpeas

Snack 2:
2 rye crispbreads with cashew nut butter

Dinner:
150g salmon (or other oily fish) or turkey with 120g spinach, 120g peppers and 75g brown rice

 Vegetarian option: 10 Quorn™ meatballs with 100g cauliflower, 100g purple sprouting broccoli and 75g brown rice;

2-3 tbsp full-fat probiotic yoghurt with 20 blueberries and 2 tbsp mixed seeds

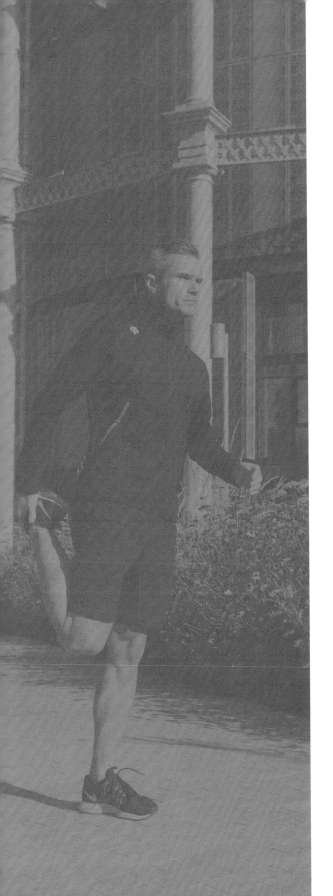

Day
42

Two weeks to go until the end of the programme. You will definitely have noticed significant changes to your body by now. But how are your energy levels and your mood? And what about your libido? My guess is that they have all improved over the last six weeks.

Fasting Diet Plan

Meal 1:
porridge made with 2 tbsp oats with a handful of berries

Meal 2:
150g protein (lean meat, fish or tofu); mixed salad containing 80g lettuce, 100g kale or spinach and 100g of two other raw vegetables, chopped or grated

Meal 3:
150g protein (lean meat, fish or tofu); mixed salad containing 80g lettuce, 100g kale or spinach and 100g of two other raw vegetables, chopped or grated

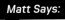

Matt Says:

Reward yourself by looking in the mirror today and acknowledging your changing body shape

Day 43

Nobody has the time to spend hours in the gym every day, which is why I don't advocate wasting your time repping out 100 bicep curls. Make your workouts count and 'lift heavy' is our rule.

➡ Mobility and activation drills (see pages 100–103)

➡ Main workout

Strength focus: 5 sets

1. Squat
No. of reps: 5
Sets: 5
Tempo: 2:0:2:0
(eccentric slow)
Rest: 90 secs

Superset 1: 4 sets

1. Incline Dumbbell Press
No. of reps: 10
Tempo: 1:0:3:0
(eccentric slow)
Rest: None

2. Single Arm Row
No. of reps: 10
Tempo: 1:0:3:0
(eccentric slow)
Rest: 60 secs

Superset 2: 4 sets

1. Shoulder Press
No. of reps: 10
Tempo: 1:0:3:0
Rest: None

2. Bicep Curl
No. of reps: 10
Tempo: 1:0:3:0
(eccentric slow)
Rest: None

Superset 3: 4 sets

1. Shoulder Press
No. of reps: 10
Tempo: 1:0:3:0
Rest: None

2. Hammer Curl
No. of reps: 10
Tempo: 1:0:3:0
Rest: 60 secs

➡ Choose a finisher routine (1, 2 or 3)

Diet Plan

Breakfast:
warm lemon water; Mexican eggs (huevos rancheros) made with 3 eggs, 1 chopped small onion, 1 pepper, 2 tbsp cannellini beans, 1–2 tbsp chopped tomatoes and Tabasco®

Snack 1:
unlimited vegetable crudités (carrots, cauliflower and broccoli) and 2 tbsp beetroot hummus

Lunch:
150g chicken with 50g edamame beans, 1 tbsp crushed peanuts, 100g quinoa and 100g brown rice

 Vegetarian option: 300g mixed salad with 150g tofu, hemp and flaxseeds, 15 pistachios and 3 tbsp chickpeas

Snack:
protein shake (20g whey, 150ml skimmed milk, 50g spinach and 2 tsp almond butter)

Dinner:
150g veal, venison, duck or ostrich (dry cooked in non-stick pan) with 120g broccoli, 1 medium sweet potato and 50–70g chickpeas

 Vegetarian option: cauliflower egg-fried rice with 120g broccoli and 120g kale

2 tbsp quark with 2 tsp honey and a few strawberries

Day 44

Make today a kale-rich day. It really is the ultimate superfood. Pack your plate with this leafy green for less than 50 calories per large serving and you will also be topping up on some important vitamins and minerals. Calorie for calorie, kale has more iron than beef and more calcium than milk, and tonnes of cancer-fighting vitamin K.

Fasting Diet Plan

Meal 1:
porridge made with 2 tbsp oats with a handful of berries

Meal 2:
150g protein (lean meat, fish or tofu); mixed salad containing 80g lettuce, 100g kale or spinach and 100g of two other raw vegetables, chopped or grated

Meal 3:
150g protein (lean meat, fish or tofu); mixed salad containing 80g lettuce, 100g kale or spinach and 100g of two other raw vegetables, chopped or grated

Matt Says:

My diet plan is as much about longevity and wellness as it is about weight

Day 45

Try to make your exercises fluid and with a good tempo – by that I mean don't start at a fast and furious pace only to slow at the end of a set.

➡ Mobility and activation drills (see pages 100–103)

➡ Main workout

Group 1: 3 sets

1. Lateral Lunge with Heel Touch
No. of reps: 10 each leg
Tempo: explosive
Rest: 30 secs

2. Alternating Spiderman
No. of reps: 30
Tempo: controlled
Rest: 30 secs

3. Burpee
No. of reps: 5
Tempo: explosive
Rest: 30 secs

4. Walking Lunge
No. of reps: 15 steps (forwards)
Tempo: controlled
Rest: 30 secs

5. Raised Plank with Shoulder Touch
No. of reps: 20-30
Tempo: controlled
Rest: 30 secs

6. Walking Lunge
No. of reps: 15 steps (backwards)
Tempo: controlled
Rest: 30 secs

7. Raised Plank with Shoulder Touch
No. of reps: 20-30
Tempo: controlled
Rest: 30 secs

Group 2: 3 sets

1. Box Jump (see page 128)
No. of reps: 15
Tempo: explosive
Rest: 30 secs

2. Single Leg Glute Bridge
No. of reps: 15 each leg
Tempo: controlled
Rest: 30 secs

3. Raised Press-up
No. of reps: to failure
Tempo: controlled
Rest: 30 secs

4. Squat Thrust
No. of reps: 10-20
Tempo: explosive
Rest: 30 secs

Diet Plan

Breakfast:
warm lemon water; 150g Greek yoghurt with 1 tsp cashew nut butter and 15 blueberries

Snack 1:
handful of almonds and raisins

Lunch:
150g sliced turkey or tofu with 50g butter beans, 1 small red onion, 1-2 tomatoes, 4 new potatoes; dressing (olive oil, tarragon and basil)

Snack 2:
apple with 3 tsp almond butter

Dinner:
tofu and vegetable patties made with 100g tofu and 100g spinach; 1 medium sweet potato and some celeriac; 25g dark chocolate

Phase Four

By Phase Four your muscle adaptation should be really evident and the progressive resistance increase should mean that you are now moving a large amount of weight during every workout.

The main change in Phase Four is the addition of drop sets. The aim here is to move as much weight as possible for the required exercise. Then, once you have created fatigue without rest, drop the weight and perform the same exercise again to double-overload the muscle group.

Phase One

Phase Two

Phase Three

Phase Four

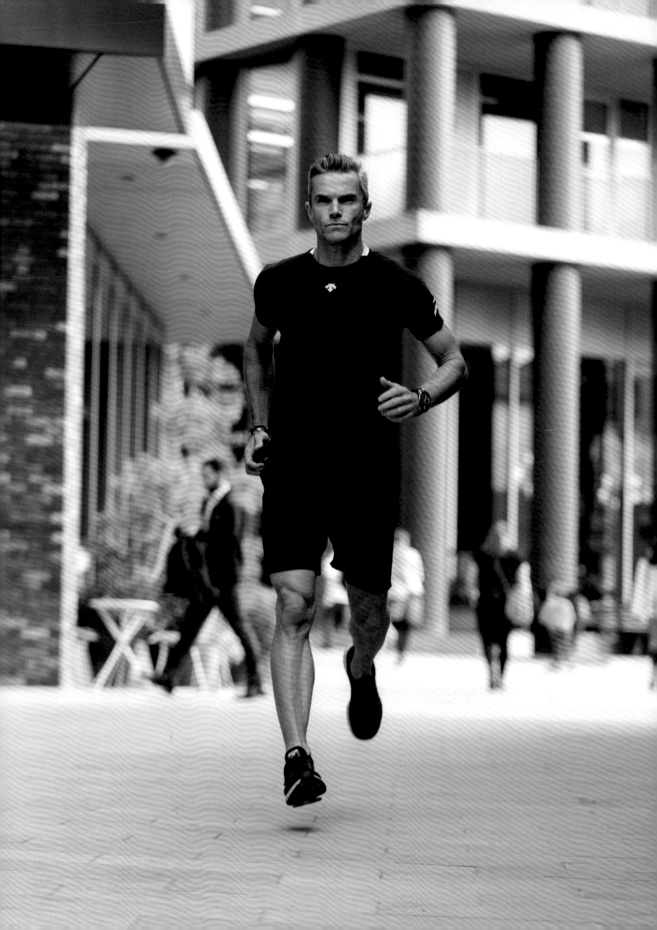

Day 46

You are into the final phase of your programme and deserve to feel a real sense of accomplishment. But don't rest on your laurels. You are not at the finish line yet. Keep focused and keep energised by eating and sleeping well – make the most of your rest day.

Diet Plan

Breakfast:
4 tbsp nut granola with 100g fat-free Greek yoghurt, 20g protein powder, 15 blueberries and 10 raspberries

Snack 1:
cup of green tea

Lunch:
salad made with 100g prawns or vegetarian cheese, ¼ cucumber, 40g goat's cheese, 10 walnuts, 10 olives, 10 cherry tomatoes and 40g beetroot

Snack 2:
60g protein bar

Dinner:
stir-fry with 200g vegetables, 100g chicken or tofu and a handful of peanuts; 150g low-fat Greek yoghurt with raspberries

Matt Says:

Revisit your sleep ritual tonight. Make sure you are doing everything you can to optimise your night recovery

Almonds are on today's menu, and for good reason. In one study [11], 82 people with elevated LDL cholesterol followed a cholesterol-lowering diet that included either 1.5 oz of almonds or a muffin with a similar number of calories (the control diet) for 6 weeks. They then swapped to eat the opposite diet for a further 6 weeks. Compared with the control diet, the almond diet led to a favourable distribution of beneficial HDL cholesterol.

➡ Mobility and activation drills (see pages 100–103)

➡ Main workout

Strength focus: 6 sets

1. Trap Bar Deadlift
No. of reps: 10, 5, 3, 1, 3, 5
Tempo: 1:0:3:0
Rest: 2 mins

Superset 1: 4 sets

1. Bench Press
No. of reps: 10
Tempo: 3:0:1:0
Rest: None

2. Pull-up
No. of reps: to failure
Tempo: controlled
Rest: 60 secs

Superset 2: 4 sets

1. Weighted Split Squat
No. of reps: 10
Tempo: 2:0:2:0
Rest: None

2. Nordic Curl
No. of reps: 10
Tempo: slow eccentric
Rest: 60 secs

Superset 3: 4 sets

1. Press-up
No. of reps: to failure
Tempo: 1:0:1:0
Rest: None

2. Lat Pulldown
No. of reps: 10
Tempo: 2:0:2:0
Rest: 60 secs

➡ Choose a finisher routine (1, 2 or 3)

Diet Plan

Breakfast:
warm lemon water; porridge made with 2 tbsp oats with a handful each of raspberries and blueberries

Snack 1:
protein smoothie (20g protein powder, 150ml semi-skimmed milk, ½ banana, 2 tbsp oats and 2 tsp almond butter)

Lunch:
150g cottage cheese with avocado, pearl barley, raw, thinly sliced red cabbage, a handful of chopped kale and 50g kidney beans

Snack 2:
a handful of almonds and raisins

Dinner:
chilli with 150g beef or Quorn™ mince, 80g kidney beans, a handful of spring greens and 120g brown rice; 25g dark chocolate

**Day
48**

It's rest day today so make the most of it. Plan something relaxing and rewarding such as a sports massage or a yoga class. Yoga is fantastic for addressing holistic aspects of life and enhancing relaxation. I've become a fan of it as an adjunct to my own training so do recommend you try it.

Diet Plan

Breakfast:
3 scrambled eggs with ½ an avocado and a pinch of zaatar

Snack 1:
apple with 3 tsp almond butter

Lunch:
100g mussels with 100g new potatoes and a rocket salad

(V) *Vegetarian option:* bowl of beetroot soup with 1 tbsp Greek yoghurt; protein shake (40g protein powder, 50g spinach and 1 tbsp almond butter)

Snack 2:
unlimited crudités (carrots, cauliflower and broccoli) with 2 tbsp beetroot hummus

Dinner:
150g baked, steamed or poached salmon or trout with 120g kale and 120g celeriac

(V) *Vegetarian option:* green Thai curry with 180g seitan and 120g Tenderstem® broccoli

25g dark chocolate

Day 49

A week to go until your 8-week programme is completed. Beyond that I hope you will be sticking with your new-found regimen and making the lifestyle adaptations you have adopted into permanent changes to your approach to exercise, diet and daily life.

➡ **Mobility and activation drills** (see pages 100–103)

➡ **Main workout**

Strength focus:

1. Squat
No. of reps: 8, 10-15
Sets: 5
Tempo: 2:0:2:0
Rest: 90-120 secs

Superset 1:
4 sets

1. Incline Dumbbell Press
No. of reps: 8, 10-15
Tempo: 1:0:2:0
Rest: None

2. Single Arm Row
No. of reps: 8, 10-15
Tempo: 1:0:2:0
Rest: 60 secs

Superset 2:
4 sets

1. Shoulder Press
No. of reps: 10
Tempo: 1:0:3:0
Rest: None

2. Bicep Curl
No. of reps: 10
Tempo: 2:0:3:0
(eccentric slow)
Rest: 60 secs

Superset 3:
4 sets

1. Lateral Raise
No. of reps: 10
Tempo: 2:0:2:0
Rest: None

2. Hammer Curl
No. of reps: 10
Tempo: 1:0:3:0
Rest: 60 secs

➡ **Choose a finisher routine** (1, 2 or 3)

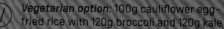

Diet Plan

Breakfast:
warm lemon water; 150g Greek yoghurt with 1 tsp cashew nut butter and 15 blueberries

Snack 1:
a handful of almonds and raisins

Lunch:
150g salmon with 50g edamame beans, 1 tbsp crushed peanuts, 100g quinoa and 100g brown rice

(V) *Vegetarian option:* 300g mixed salad with 150g tofu, hemp and flaxseeds, 15 pistachios and 3 tbsp chickpeas

Snack 2:
protein shake (20g whey, 150ml skimmed milk, 50g spinach and 2 tsp almond butter)

Dinner:
150g veal, venison, duck or ostrich (dry cooked in non-stick pan) with 120g broccoli, 1 medium sweet potato and 50-70g chickpeas

(V) *Vegetarian option:* 100g cauliflower egg-fried rice with 120g broccoli and 120g kale

25g dark chocolate

Day
50

You've been eating a lot of porridge over the last few weeks and probably know already that it is an excellent source of fibre and fills you up for hours on end. But, consumed on a regular basis, it's also a key to longevity. A major study by Harvard University researchers [12] involving 100,000 people and over a period of more than 14 years found that whole grains, including porridge, reduce the risk of dying from heart disease.

Fasting Diet Plan

Meal 1:
porridge made with 2 tbsp oats with a handful of berries

Meal 2:
150g protein (lean meat, fish or tofu); mixed salad containing 80g lettuce, 100g kale or spinach and 100g of two other raw vegetables, chopped or grated

Meal 3:
150g protein (lean meat, fish or tofu); mixed salad containing 80g lettuce, 100g kale or spinach and 100g of two other raw vegetables, chopped or grated

Day 51

Burpees are a tough exercise as you have no doubt discovered by now, but they bring endless benefits with the effort entailed. They don't just work your whole body, they require all your muscles to work in unison as you perform the movement and are an important exercise in helping to develop strength, power, agility, and coordination.

➡ **Mobility and activation drills** (see pages 100–103)

➡ **Main workout**

Group 1: 3 sets

1. Lateral Lunge with Heel Touch
No. of reps: 10 each leg
Tempo: explosive
Rest: 30 secs

2. Alternating Spiderman
No. of reps: 30
Tempo: controlled
Rest: 30 secs

3. Burpee
No. of reps: 5
Tempo: explosive
Rest: 30 secs

4. Walking Lunge
No. of reps: 15 steps (forwards)
Tempo: controlled
Rest: 30 secs

5. Raised Plank with Shoulder Touch
No. of reps: 20-30
Tempo: controlled
Rest: 30 secs

6. Walking Lunge
No. of reps: 15 steps (backwards)
Tempo: controlled
Rest: 30 secs

7. Raised Plank with Forward Reach
No. of reps: 20-30
Tempo: controlled
Rest: 30 secs

Group 2: 3 sets

1. Box Jump (see page 128)
No. of reps: 15
Tempo: explosive
Rest: 30 secs

2. Single Leg Glute Bridge
No. of reps: 15 each leg
Tempo: controlled
Rest: 30 secs

3. Raised Press-up
No. of reps: to failure
Tempo: controlled
Rest: 30 secs

4. Squat Thrust
No. of reps: 10-20
Tempo: explosive
Rest: 30 secs

Diet Plan

Breakfast:
warm lemon water; 150g Greek yoghurt with 1 tsp cashew nut butter and 15 blueberries

Snack 1:
a handful of almonds and raisins

Lunch:
150g chicken with 50g edamame beans, 1 tbsp crushed peanuts, 100g quinoa and 100g cooked rice

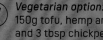 *Vegetarian option:* 300g mixed salad with 150g tofu, hemp and flaxseeds, 15 pistachios and 3 tbsp chickpeas

Snack 2:
2 rye crispbreads with cashew nut butter

Dinner:
150g salmon (or other oily fish) with 120g spinach and 120g peppers

 Vegetarian option: 10 Quorn™ meatballs with 100g cauliflower and 100g purple sprouting broccoli

150g full-fat probiotic yoghurt with 20 blueberries and 2 tbsp mixed seeds

**Day
52**

My betting is that at the start of this programme you might have struggled with the prospect of fasting for two days a week. Now? I imagine it is beginning to slip seamlessly into your routine. It helps that your diet on the non-fasting days is replete with nutrients and energy and that you have been cutting out processed and refined foods that trigger hunger pangs and cravings. Well done for getting here.

Fasting Diet Plan

Meal 1:
porridge made with 2 tbsp oats with a handful of berries

Meal 2:
150g protein (lean meat, fish or tofu); mixed salad containing 80g lettuce, 100g kale or spinach and 100g of two other raw vegetables, chopped or grated

Meal 3:
150g protein (lean meat, fish or tofu); mixed salad containing 80g lettuce, 100g kale or spinach and 100g of two other raw vegetables, chopped or grated

Matt Says:

Porridge has been shown to sustain energy levels better than commercial sports drinks

Day 53

If you are feeling tired, I would like you to focus your attention on mobility and core drills before the main session today. They encompass many aspects of physical development and my clients are often surprised at the difference these drills make to their overall progress.

Mobility and activation drills (see pages 100–103)

Main workout

Strength focus:
6 sets

1. Trap Bar Deadlift
No. of reps: 10, 5, 3, 1, 3, 5
Tempo: 1:0:3:0
Rest: 2 mins

Superset 2:
4 sets

1. Bench Press
No. of reps: 10
Tempo: 3:0:1:0
Rest: None

2. Pull-up
No. of reps: to failure
Tempo: controlled
Rest: 60 secs

Superset 3:
4 sets

1. Weighted Split Squat
No. of reps: 10
Tempo: 2:0:2:0
Rest: None

2. Nordic Curl
No. of reps: 10
Tempo: slow eccentric
Rest: 60 secs

Superset 4:
4 sets

1. Press-up
No. of reps: to failure
Tempo: 1:0:1:0
Rest: None

2. Lat pulldown
No. of reps: 10
Tempo: 2:0:2:0
Rest: 60 secs

Choose a finisher routine (1, 2 or 3)

Diet Plan

Breakfast:
warm lemon water; 3-egg omelette with 150g spinach and 100g mushrooms; small glass of grapefruit juice

Snack 1:
4 rice cakes and 2 tbsp hummus

Lunch:
150g crab meat with 3-4 florets of broccoli, 1 medium sweet potato, 50g of feta cheese and 200g brown rice

 Vegetarian option: 300g mixed salad tossed with 150g tofu and 70g feta; cup of green tea

Snack 2:
protein smoothie (20g whey, a handful of spinach, 1 pear, 1–2 sticks celery and 3–4 florets of broccoli)

Dinner:
150g lean steak (dry cooked in grill or non-stick pan) with 120g broad beans, 120g cabbage and 120g kidney beans

(V) *Vegetarian option:* 2 Quorn™ burgers with 120g kale, 120g courgette and 120g broccoli

2-3 tbsp quark with 2 tsp honey and a few strawberries

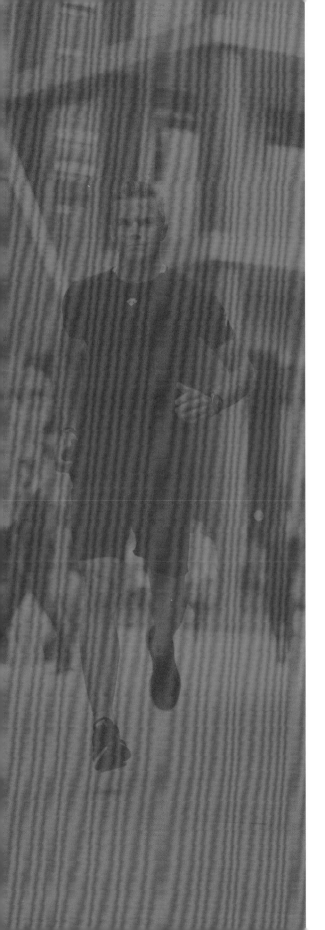

Day 54

Spend today taking a well-earned break. If you really feel the need to do something, go for a walk in a park, take a cycle ride or head to a spa for a relaxing and rejuvenating sauna.

Diet Plan

Breakfast:
warm lemon water; frittata made with 3 eggs, 1 tomato, 50-75g mushrooms, a handful of spinach and 20g cheddar cheese

Snack 1:
100g fat free Greek yoghurt, 20g whey powder and 30g mixed berries

Lunch:
100g nut roast with 100g parsnips and 120g broccoli

Snack 2:
4 rice cakes and 2 tbsp hummus

Dinner:
150g steak (dry-cooked in non-stick pan) or non-meat alternative with 100g cabbage and 100g broad beans; 2 kiwi fruits

Matt Says:

Keep tabs on your stress levels – don't allow them to spiral out of control

Day 55

This is the last day you are going to work really hard before celebrating your achievements tomorrow. I want you to test yourself to see just how far you have come. Flick back in that training diary before starting your session and then wallow in your accomplishments.

➡ Mobility and activation drills (see pages 100–103)

➡ Main workout

Strength focus: 6 sets

1. Bench Press
No. of reps: 8, 10-15
Lift 8 at max, then immediately take 40% weight off and perform a further 10-15 reps
Tempo: 3:0:1:0
Rest: 90-120 secs

Superset 2: 4 sets

1. Lateral Lunge
No. of reps: 10
Tempo: 3:0:1:0
Rest: None

2. Single Leg Deadlift
No. of reps: 10
Tempo: 3:0:1:0
Rest: 60 secs

Superset 3: 4 sets

1. Dumbbell Press
No. of reps: 10
Tempo: 4:0:1:0
Rest: None

2. Dumbbell Pullover
No. of reps: 10
Tempo: 4:0:1:0
Rest: 60 secs

Superset 4: 4 sets

1. Face Pull
No. of reps: 10
Tempo: 3:0:1:0
Rest: None

2. Triceps Push Down
No. of reps: 10
Tempo: 3:0:1:0
Rest: 60 secs

Diet Plan

Breakfast:
warm lemon water; 3-egg omelette with 150g spinach and 100g mushrooms; small glass of grapefruit juice

Snack 1:
4 rice cakes and 2 tbsp hummus

Lunch:
150g chicken with 50g edamame beans, 1 tbsp crushed peanuts and 100g quinoa

 Vegetarian option: 300g mixed salad with 150g tofu, hemp and flaxseeds, 15 pistachios and 3 tbsp chickpeas

Snack 2:
2 rye crispbreads with cashew nut butter

Dinner:
10 lean meat or Quorn™ meatballs with 100g cauliflower, 100g purple sprouting broccoli and 50g chickpeas; 150g probiotic yoghurt with 20 blueberries and 2 tbsp mixed seeds

Day 56

You made it! Congratulations. This is what all of the hard work has been about – the chance to achieve this goal. After eight weeks on the programme you must look and feel fantastic. Your weight has dropped, your energy levels and libido have soared and you feel like a younger, fitter and stronger version of your former self. Long may it continue, so make sure you read the What's Next chapter of this book (page 196).

Diet Plan

Breakfast:
warm lemon water; porridge made with 2 tbsp oats with a handful each of raspberries and blueberries

Snack 1:
a handful of almonds and raisins

Lunch:
300g mixed salad with 150g tofu, hemp and flaxseeds, 15 pistachios and 3 tbsp chickpeas

Snack 2:
2 tbsp red pepper dip with celery

Dinner:
150g steak or non-meat steak, burger or meatball with 100g cabbage, 100g broad beans and 10 new potatoes; 2 tbsp quark with 2 tsp honey and a few raspberries

Matt Says:

You have achieved something remarkable. It's never easy to set about changing the way we live and yet you have succeeded. Full respect.

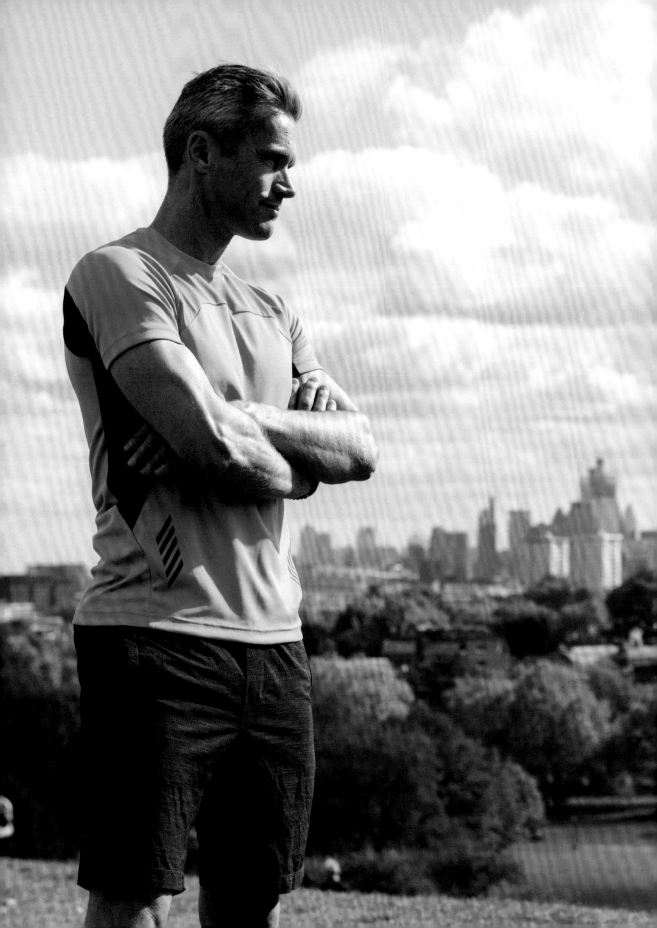

Chapter Twelve

What Next?

You have completed the 8-week plan and, I hope, are enjoying the results you see and feel. However, in many ways this is the beginning of a lifelong approach to living well. It can be daunting to think too far ahead, which is why I have created simple steps for you to follow so that the good work is not undone. It will be easier than you might think.

Looking Ahead

Your future can be one that is rewarding and energising in equal measure. By now you will realise that it is possible to look and feel ten or even 20 years younger. Long may it continue

Congratulations for completing the programme. My guess is that you are feeling and looking so much better than you did eight weeks ago. But it shouldn't end here. In many ways, this is the beginning – of a life more fulfilled and more fulfilling. What I don't want is for you to go back to your old habits, but neither do I want you to continue aimlessly with no sense of direction. It is all too easy to just keep going, adding more intensity and not realising what you have achieved and how you can maintain that improvement and set new goals without it taking over your entire life. Here's my advice about what to do next:

Take a breath and look at what you have achieved

The most important thing to do when you come to the end of an intensive programme, like this, is to take a second to review your progress. Answer the questions below as honestly as you can, making notes if you feel the need:

→ How do you feel?
→ How do you look?
→ How hard was it?
→ How easy was it to fit into normal life? (This will shape how, and if, you can maintain what you have achieved.)
→ What was the hardest part of the programme?

Take a week off

You deserve it! You have just worked hard for eight weeks and need some time to recover. Don't go crazy by eating too unhealthily and do exercise if you feel like it. Just don't be too strict on yourself.

Keep up with the diet

If the amount of time and effort that this programme has taken felt achievable, the way forward for you is really quite simple. The diet plan that we have worked on in this programme is one that can be carried forward and the more you get used to it the easier your routine becomes.

Outside of the programme you will probably have a couple of cheat days in the week where you are not so strict with your diet. However, I would really encourage you to maintain at least one if not two fast days as these will offset any cheat days that you are likely to have. Don't have cheat days and then feel guilty, accept that it happens and that it is a good thing to let your hair down every now and again. Just make sure that you have your back-up procedures that keep you on the right path and keep you fit, strong and healthy.

Keep pushing yourself

From a training point of view you need to keep on improving your strength, you need to focus on maintaining the hypertrophy element to our training and you need to make sure that the metabolic training component is there. You also need to make sure that you keep on pushing the body that little bit harder and making sure that you introduce new elements to how you train. If the body gets too used to a style of training, it becomes lazy.

One of the key factors to always be aware of is your training weight volume. This is the total amount of weight that you push or pull. On the whole, with all my lifts I try to make sure that I always keep on increasing my training weight volume. If I was doing 5 sets of 5 reps at 100kg per rep, that would give me a total weight pushed of 2500kg. Therefore, in 2 weeks' time I would need to be lifting more than 2500kg in total on that one movement. What I like about using training volume is that I know that I am working harder each time I go in the gym. I know that the total amount I am pushing is going up and I therefore know that my 1 rep max – the maximum amount of weight I can lift in a single attempt - will be improving.

It is important to always have clear markers to understand your progression. This can be volume on each particular exercise or volume of your whole workout.

Stick to the programme as much as you can

If you found that the effort required over the last eight weeks was too much, it is not the end of the world. The programme was a controlled effort that guided you in the right direction, where you managed to achieve some great results and feel good about yourself. However, take a moment to work out what percentage of the programme you could actually manage to fit into your lifestyle.

What I have outlined in this programme is really what is required to feel fit, strong, healthy and mobile for years. Any less than this and you have to ask yourself how much of a priority a healthy long life really is to you. We can all use the excuse of life being busy or work being stressful, but this is the essence of what we are talking about: if you can't find the time to keep yourself fit and healthy, why are you doing what you are doing? Waiting for the day when life is less stressful and you have more time to think about eating and exercise will be too late.

For you, the following rules apply:

→ Aim to have more control and routine to what you eat and drink.
→ Allow yourself cheat days, but don't let days become weeks.
→ Maintain the strength element to whatever exercise you do in the week. Most of our ageing comes from a lack of muscle and the skeletal control that comes with that. Just doing some cardio a couple of times per week will not have enough of this effect.
→ Aim for consistency. Don't fit in exercise when you can. Plan it, don't move it for something else and make it your key priority. Make you your key priority. The fitter you are, the better you are for all around you.
→ Find a training buddy. Study after study has shown how we achieve greater sustained goals if we share the workload and share the success.

In the three decades I have been training people there is nothing that gives me greater pleasure than seeing the growth in confidence and self-worth that comes with being fit and healthy. This positive feeling threads itself into social life, work life and family life and I have seen so many people make huge positive changes to their lives because they felt better about themselves. It can do this for anyone and I encourage you to embrace it.

→ Terminology Explained

There's a lot of complex jargon when it comes to diet and fitness. It's easy to get bewildered and confused by it, which is why I have provided simple explanations for some of the terms I've used.

Your workouts

Reps: (Short for 'repetitions') The number of times you consecutively perform a specific exercise.

Sets: The number of cycles of reps you complete with a rest between each.

Supersets: Two different exercise sets performed without a break. Supersetting is a highly effective way to achieve muscle overload and work opposing muscles in quick succession via pairs of exercises. It's time-efficient as you don't need to stop for long bouts of recovery between exercises. It works because it keeps the intensity high and as one side of the body works hard, the other rests.

Overloading: The underlying principle of any exercise programme. Essentially it means that you are working your muscles outside of their comfort zone and pushing your body to new levels of exertion. As a consequence, your muscles are forced to work harder and to respond and adapt to the pressures placed upon them in a positive way.

Activation drills: A series of pre-workout exercises designed to fire up the secondary muscles that are so important in large movements.

Mobility drills: A series of pre-workout drills that aim to improve mobility all over the body. Most entail using foam rollers and other aids.

Compound training: A way of exercising that entails isolating specific muscles and then adding exercises for other supporting muscles as that muscle weakens.

Delayed Onset Muscle Soreness (DOMS): The aching feeling you get 48–72 hours after a session. Some DOMS is to be expected, but if you increase your sets and reps too aggressively, you can almost guarantee that you will experience a high level of DOMS. There's a fine line between acceptable and excessive DOMS that limits training intensity, frequency and athletic performance. The rule is not to progress too quickly.

Concentric movement: The phase when the muscle shortens in length, e.g. when lifting a weight.

Eccentric movement: The phase when the muscle lengthens, e.g. when you lower a weight back to the starting position.

Eccentric slow: Instruction to perform the eccentric phase of a movement slowly. This enhances hypertrophy, the ability to build lean muscle.

Load-bearing exercise: Exercise where your body supports its own weight, having to work against gravity, e.g. running, jumping, weight training, etc. This is good for improving bone strength.

Maximise reps: Instruction to push yourself as hard as possible for every rep, stopping just before the point when you feel your technique might falter, or you feel like you might fail on the next rep.

Maximum heart rate (MHR): The number of beats of your heart in 1 minute when working at maximum effort.

Resting heart rate (RHR): The number of beats of your heart in 1 minute when you are at complete rest, i.e. sitting or lying down.

Your body

Androgens: Male sex hormones

Anabolic: Relating to the building of molecules and muscle cells

Catabolic: Relating to the breakdown of molecules and muscle cells

Human growth hormone (HGH): The naturally occurring growth hormone in humans that stimulates growth, cell reproduction and cell regeneration.

Luteinising hormone: A hormone secreted by the anterior pituitary gland that stimulates the synthesis of androgen in men (and ovulation in females).

Male hypogonadism: A clinical condition where the body doesn't produce enough testosterone and/or has an impaired ability to produce sperm.

Oestrogen: A group of hormones known as 'female hormones' that stimulates the development and maintenance of female sexual characteristics. They are also present in the male body.

Testosterone: A steroid hormone that stimulates development of male sexual characteristics. Produced mainly in the testes, but also in the adrenal cortex. It is also present in the female body.

Telomeres: Area of DNA found at the ends of the chromosomes which protect against cell damage. Telomere length shortens with age.

Neurogenesis: The process by which new neurons are formed in the brain.

Microbiome (microbiota): The vast ecosystem of bacteria, fungi and viruses that inhabits the human body and specifically the gut. Your body is home to about 100 trillion bacteria and other microbes, collectively known as microbiota.

Insulin-like growth factor-1 (IGF-1): A hormone that, along with human growth hormone (HGH), helps promote normal bone and tissue growth and development.

Hypertrophy: The growth and increase in size of muscle cells as a result of weight training and physical exercise.

Overtraining: Often the result of 'overreaching' in sessions and inadequate recovery between exercise sessions. Symptoms include disrupted sleep, more illness and injury and a plateau or drop in fitness.

Cryotherapy: The use of cold temperatures to accelerate muscle recovery and repair, e.g. ice baths used by elite athletes following a hard training session or event.

Creatine kinase: An important enzyme in muscle tissue that has a proven anti-ageing effect and is an indicator of muscle damage.

Heart Rate Variability (HRV): Measure of the variation in time between each heartbeat. A low HRV is linked to low mood, an increased risk of death and cardiovascular disease.

Glutes: The muscles in the buttocks and hip area that are used to move the legs backwards

Hip flexor: The muscles positioned at the top of the hip. They can become stiff and tight through chronic sitting and are important for movements such as bringing the knee towards the chest.

Lats (latissimus dorsi): The largest muscle of the back, used in any pulling motion.

Pecs: The pectoral muscles in the chest area, used for pushing movements.

Moobs (man boobs): Fatty deposits that appear in the chest area of men of and are due to an increase in the production of oestrogen in the body.

Core: Group of muscles that are responsible for the stabilisation of the spine. They lie deep within your torso and are attached to the spine and pelvis. They include the deeply embedded transversus abdominis that is hard to target with regular exercise, and the muscles of the pelvic floor as well as the muscles at the side of the waist – called the obliques.

Fascia: The dense, fibrous connective tissue around the body that surrounds all muscles and bones.

Your nutrition

Branched Chain Amino acids (BCAAs): Three amino acids – leucine, isoleucine and valine – that promote muscle protein synthesis and increase muscle growth over time. They are obtained from protein-rich foods such as chicken, fish, eggs, beans, lentils, nuts and soy protein but can also be taken as a supplement.

Gamma-aminobutyric acid (GABA): An important neurotransmitter in the central nervous system. It can be taken as a supplement.

Glycaemic index: Rating system for foods containing carbohydrates, indicating how quickly it affects your blood sugar (glucose) level. Low GI foods tend to be higher in fibre and have a longer-lasting energy burst than those with a high GI.

L-glutamine: A conditionally essential amino acid. It can be taken as a supplement.

5-hydroxytryptophan (5-HTP): Compound made naturally in the body as a by-product of the amino acid L-tryptophan. It can be taken as a supplement.

Leucine: An amino acid that enhances male hormone production. Found in cheese, soybeans, beef, chicken, pork, nuts, seeds, fish and seafood, but can also be taken as a supplement.

D-Aspartic acid: An amino acid that plays a role in increasing testosterone production. Can be taken as a supplement.

Oyster body extract: The dried and powdered meat of an oyster, it is rich in zinc, known to be essential for testosterone production. It can be taken as a supplement.

References

Chapter 1: The Science

1. Travison, T.G. et al., 'A Population-Level Decline in Serum Testosterone Levels in American Men', *Journal of Clinical Endocrinology & Metabolism*, 92/1 (2007), 196–202

2. Andersson, A.M. et al., 'Secular Decline in Male Testosterone and Sex Hormone Binding Globulin Serum Levels in Danish Population Surveys', *Journal of Clinical Endocrinology & Metabolism*, 92/12 (2007), 4696–4705

3. Peterson, M.D. et al., 'Testosterone Deficiency, Weakness, and Multimorbidity in Men', *Scientific Reports*, 8/1 (2018)

4. Westley, C.J. et al., 'High Rates of Depression and Depressive Symptoms among Men Referred for Borderline Testosterone Levels', *Journal of Sexual Medicine*, 12/8 (2015), 1753–60

5. Finkelstein, J.S. et al., 'Gonadal Steroids and Body Composition, Strength, and Sexual Function in Men', *New England Journal of Medicine*, 369 (2013), 1011–1022

6. Leproult, R. and Van Cauter, E., 'Effect of 1 Week of Sleep Restriction on Testosterone Levels in Young Healthy Men', *Journal of American Medical Association*, 305/21 (2011), 2173–4

7. McLaughlin, M.A. et al.,'Low Serum Testosterone is Associated with Obstructive Sleep Apnea in Middle Aged Men', *Journal of Urology*, 187/4 (2012), e561

8. Zitzmann, M., 'Testosterone and the Brain', *Aging Male*, 9/4 (2006), 195–9

9. Moffat, S.D. et al., 'Free Testosterone and Risk for Alzheimer Disease in Older Men', *Neurology*, 62/2 (2004), 188–93

10. Anawalt, B.D., 'Testosterone and the Brain' in Jones, H., *Testosterone Deficiency in Men 2ⁿᵈ Edition* (Oxford, 2012; chapter 13)

11. Loprinzi, P.D. et al., 'Movement-Based Behaviors and Leukocyte Telomere Length among US Adults', *Medicine and Science in Sports and Exercise*, 47/11 (2015), 2347–52

12. Craig, B.W. et al., 'Effects of Progressive Resistance Training on Growth Hormone and Testosterone Levels in Young and Elderly Subjects', *Mechanisms of Aging and Development*, 49/2 (1989), 159–169

13. Morton, R.W. et al., 'Neither Load nor Systemic Hormones Determine Resistance Training-Mediated Hypertrophy or Strength Gains in Resistance-Trained Young Men', *Journal of Applied Physiology*, 121/1 (2016), 129–138

14. Stokes, K.A. et al., 'The Time Course of the Human Growth Hormone Response to a 6s and a 30s Cycle Ergometer Sprint', *Journal of Sports Science*, 20/6 (2002), 487–94

15. Pollock, R.D. et al., 'Properties of the Vastus Lateralis Muscle in Relation to Age and Physiological Function in Master Cyclists Aged 55–79 years', *Aging Cell*, 17/2 (2018), e12735

16. Duggal, N.A. et al., 'Major Features of Immunesenescence, including Reduced Thymic Output, are Ameliorated by High Levels of Physical Activity in Adulthood', *Aging Cell*, 17/2 (2018), e12750

17. Hackney, A.C. and Aggon, E., 'Chronic Low Testosterone Levels in Endurance Trained Men: The Exercise-Hypogonadal Male Condition', *Journal of Biochemistry and Physiology*, 1/1 (2018), 103

18. Crouse, L., 'His Strength Sapped, Top Marathoner Ryan Hall Decides to Stop', *New York Times* (Jan 15, 2016)

19. Steves, C.J. et al., 'Kicking Back Cognitive Ageing: Leg Power Predicts Cognitive Ageing after Ten Years in Older Female Twins', *Gerontology*, 62/2 (2016), 138–149

20. Mavros, Y. et al., 'Mediation of Cognitive Function Improvements by Strength Gains After Resistance Training in Older Adults with Mild Cognitive Impairment: Outcomes of the Study of Mental and Resistance Training', *Journal of the American Geriatrics Society*, 65/3 (2016), 550–559

21. Adami, R. et al., 'Reduction of Movement in Neurological Diseases: Effects on Neural Stem Cells Characteristics', *Frontiers in Neuroscience*, 12 (2018), 336

Chapter 3: Nutrition

1. Sierksma, A. et al., 'Effect of Moderate Alcohol Consumption on Plasma Dehydroepiandrosterone Sulfate, Testosterone, and Estradiol Levels in Middle-Aged men and Postmenopausal Women: a Diet-Controlled Intervention Study', *Alcoholism Clinical & Experimental Research*, 28/5 (2004), 780–5

2. Caronia, L.M. et al., 'Abrupt Decrease in Serum Testosterone Levels after an Oral Glucose Load in Men: Implications for Screening for Hypogonadism', *Clinical Endocrinology*, 78/2 (2013), 291–6

3. Gabel, K. et al., 'Effects of 8-Hour Time Restricted Feeding on Body Weight and Metabolic Disease Risk Factors in Obese Adults: A Pilot Study', *Nutrition and Healthy Aging*, 4 (4) (2018), 345–353

4. Grube, B.J. et al., 'White Button Mushroom Phytochemicals Inhibit Aromatase Activity and Breast Cancer Cell Proliferation', *Journal of Nutrition*, 131/12 (2001), 3288–93

5. Zhang, M. et al., 'Dietary Intakes of Mushrooms and Green Tea Combine to Reduce the Risk of Breast Cancer in Chinese Women', *International Journal of Cancer*; 124/6 (2009), 1404–8

Chapter 4: Digestion

1. Haruma et al., 'Lifestyle Factors and Efficacy Of Lifestyle Interventions in Gastroesophageal Reflux Disease Patients with Functional Dyspepsia: Primary Care Perspectives From THE LEGEND Study', *Internal Medicine*, 54/7 (2015), 695–701

2. Neuman et al., 'Microbial Endocrinology: The Interplay Between The Microbiota And The Endocrine System', *FEMS Microbiology Reviews*, 39/4 (2015), 509–521

3. Spector et al., 'Gut Microbiome Diversity and High-Fibre Intake are Related to Lower Long-Term Weight Gain', *International Journal of Obesity*, 41/7 (2017), 1099–1105

4. O'Sullivan et al., 'Exercise and the Microbiota', *Gut Microbes*, 6/2 (2015), 131–136

5. Spector et al., 'Signatures of Early Frailty in the Gut Microbiota', *Genome Medicine*, 8:8 (2016)

6. Gopinath, B. et al., 'Association Between Carbohydrate Nutrition and Successful Aging Over 10 Years', *Journals of Gerontology, Series A: Biological Sciences and Medical Sciences*, 71/10 (2016), 1335–40

7. Thompson, S.V. et al., 'Effects Of Isolated Soluble Fiber Supplementation On Body Weight, Glycemia, And Insulinemia In Adults With Overweight And Obesity: A Systematic Review And Meta-Analysis Of Randomized Controlled Trials', *American Journal of Clinical Nutrition*, 106/6 (2017), 1514–1528

8. Rose, D.P. et al., 'High-Fiber Diet Reduces Serum Estrogen Concentrations in Premenopausal Women', *American Journal of Clinical Nutrition*, 54/3 (1991), 520–525

9. British Nutrition Foundation <nutrition.org.uk>

10. Schroeder, B.O. et al., 'Bifidobacteria Or Fiber Protects Against Diet-Induced Microbiota-Mediated Colonic Mucus Deterioration', *Cell Host & Microbe*, 23/1 (2017), 27–40.e7

11. Jun Zou, J. et al., 'Fiber-Mediated Nourishment Of Gut Microbiota Protects Against Diet-Induced Obesity By Restoring IL-22-Mediated Colonic Health', *Cell Host & Microbe*, 23/1 (2018), 41–53.e4

Chapter 5: Spinal Health

1. Back Care UK <www.backcare.org.uk>

2. Steffens, D. et al., 'Prevention of Low Back Pain: A Systematic Review and Meta-Analysis', *JAMA Internal Medicine*, 176/2 (2016), 199–208

3. Chartered Society of Physiotherapy <www.csp.org.uk> and <www.opinium.co.uk>

4. Kell, R.T. and Asmundson, G.J., 'A Comparison of Two Forms of Periodized Exercise Rehabilitation Programs in the Management of Chronic Nonspecific Low-Back Pain', *Journal of Strength and Conditioning Research*, 23/2 (2009), 513–23

5. Wilson F. et al., 'Ergometer Training Volume and Previous Injury Predict Back Pain in Rowing: Strategies for Injury Prevention and Rehabilitation', *British Journal of Sports Medicine*, 48 (3) (2014), 393–404

6. Cherkin, D.C. et al., 'Effect of Mindfulness-Based Stress Reduction vs Cognitive Behavioral Therapy or Usual Care on Back Pain and Functional Limitations in Adults With Chronic Low Back Pain: A Randomized Clinical Trial', *JAMA*, 315/12 (2016), 1240–1249

7. Pocari, J. et al., 'What is the Best Back Exercise?', *ACE Certified Journal* (2018)

8. McGill, S., *Back Mechanic* (2015), Backfitpro Inc.

Chapter 6: Sex and Lifestyle

1. Gettler, L.T. et al., 'Longitudinal Evidence that Fatherhood Decreases Testosterone in Human Males', *Proceedings of the National Academy of Sciences of the USA*, 108/39 (2011), 16194–9

2. Mental Health Foundation, 'Mental Health Statistics: Stress', (2018), <https://www.mentalhealth.org.uk/statistics/mental-health-statistics-stress>

3. The Physiological Society, Stress in Modern Britain (2017), <https://www.physoc.org/sites/default/files/press-release/4042-stress-modern-britain.pdf>

4. Mehta, P.H. and Josephs, R.A., 'Testosterone and Cortisol Jointly Regulate Dominance: Evidence for a Dual-Hormone Hypothesis', Hormones and Behavior, 58/5 (2010), 898-906

5. Sherman, G. D. et al., 'The Interaction of Testosterone and Cortisol is Associated with Attained Status in Male Executives', Journal of Personality and Social Psychology, 110/6 (2016), 921-929

6. Coates, J.M. and Herbert, J., 'Endogenous Steroids and Financial Risk Taking on a London Trading Floor', Proceedings of the National Academy of Sciences (PNAS), 105/16 (2008), 6167-72

7. Twal, W.O. et al., 'Yogic Breathing when Compared to Attention Control Reduces the Levels of Pro-inflammatory Biomarkers in Saliva: a Pilot Randomized Controlled Trial', BMC Complementary and Alternative Medicine, 16 (2016), 294

8. Goyal, M. 'Meditation Programs for Psychological Stress and Well-being: A Systematic Review and Meta-analysis', JAMA Internal Medicine, 174/3 (2014), 357-368

9. Jacobs, T.L. et al., 'Self-Reported Mindfulness and Cortisol During a Shamatha Meditation Retreat', Health Psychology, 32/10 (2013), 1104-9

10. Alderman, B.L. et al., 'MAP Training: Combining Meditation and Aerobic Exercise Reduces Depression and Rumination While Enhancing Synchronized Brain Activity', Translational Psychiatry 6 (2016), e726

11. Peter J. Snyder, P.J. et al., 'Effects of Testosterone Treatment in Older Men', New England Journal of Medicine, 374/7 (2016), 611

12. Cunningham, G.R. et al., 'Testosterone Treatment and Sexual Function in Older Men with Low Testosterone Levels', Journal of Clinical Endocrinology & Metabolism, 101/8 (2016), 3096-3104

13. White, J.R. et al., 'Enhanced Sexual Behavior in Exercising Men', Archives of Sexual Behaviour, 19/3 (1990), 193-209

14. van der Meij, L. et al., 'Testosterone and Cortisol Release among Spanish Soccer Fans Watching the 2010 World Cup Final', PLoS ONE, 7/4 (2012), e34814

Chapter 7: Sleep and Recovery

1. Leproult, R. and Van Cauter, E., 'Effect of 1 Week of Sleep Restriction on Testosterone Levels in Young Healthy Men', Journal of the American Medical Association, 305/21 (2011), 2173-4

2. Mah, C.D. et al., 'The Effects of Sleep Extension on the Athletic Performance of Collegiate Basketball Players', Sleep, 34/7 (2011), 943-950

3. Luke, A. et al., 'Sports-Related Injuries in Youth Athletes: Is Overscheduling a Risk Factor?', Clinical Journal of Sports Medicine, 21/4 (2011), 307-14

4. Milewski, M.D. et al., 'Chronic Lack of Sleep is Associated with Increased Sports Injuries in Adolescent Athletes', Journal of Paediatric Orthopedics, 34/2 (2014), 129-33

5. Baron, K.G. et al., 'Orthosomnia: Are Some Patients Taking the Quantified Self Too Far?', Journal of Clinical Sleep Medicine, 13/2 (2017), 351-4

6. Gottschall, J; research presented at the ACSM Annual Meeting 2018; <www.lesmills.com>

7. Gordon, J.A.III. et al., 'Comparisons in the Recovery Response from Resistance Exercise Between Young and Middle-Aged Men', Journal of Strength and Conditioning Research, 31/12 (2017), 3454-3462

8. Urrila, A.S. et al., 'Sleep Habits, Academic Performance, and the Adolescent Brain Structure', Scientific Reports, 7 (2017), article number: 41678

9. Allan, R. and Mawhinney, C., 'Is the Ice Bath Finally Melting? Cold Water Immersion Is No Greater than Active Recovery upon Local and Systemic Inflammatory Cellular Stress in Humans', Journal of Physiology, 595/6 (2017), 1857-1858

10. Hausswirth, C. et al., 'Effects of Whole-body Cryotherapy vs. Far-infrared vs. Passive Modalities on Recovery from Exercise-induced Muscle Damage in Highly-trained Runners', PLoS One, 6/12 (2011), e27749

11. Drake, C. et al., 'Caffeine Effects on Sleep Taken 0, 3, or 6 Hours Before Going to Bed', Journal of Clinical Sleep Medicine, 9/11 (2013), 1195-1200

12. Hong, K.B. et al., 'Sleep-Promoting Effects of a GABA/5-HTP Mixture: Behavioral Changes and Neuromodulation in an Invertebrate Model', Life Sciences, 150 (2016), 42-9

13. 'Theanine Increases Levels of GABA (along with Serotonin, Dopamine and Alpha Brainwave Activity) and May Reduce Mental and Physical Stress and Produce Feelings of Relaxation', Nutrients, 9/7 (2017), 777

14. Lin, H.H. et al., 'Effect of Kiwifruit Consumption on Sleep Quality in Adults with Sleep Problems', Asia Pacific Journal of Clinical Nutrition, 20/2 (2011), 169-74

15. Buccelletti, E. et al., 'Heart Rate Variability and Myocardial Infarction: Systematic Literature Review and Metanalysis', European Review for Medical and Pharmacological Sciences, 13/4 (2009), 299-307

16. Tsuji, H. et al., 'Reduced Heart Rate Variability and Mortality Risk in an Elderly Cohort: The Framingham Heart Study', Circulation, 90/2 (1994), 878-83

17. Ernst, G., 'Heart-Rate Variability — More than Heart Beats?', Front Public Health, 5 (2017), 240

18. Hautala, A.J. et al., 'Individual Differences in the Responses to Endurance and Resistance Rraining', European Journal of Applied Physiology, 96/5 (2006), 535-42

19. Vesterinen, V. et al., 'Heart Rate Variability in Prediction of Individual Adaptation to Endurance Training in Recreational Endurance Runners', Scandinavian Journal of Medicine and Science in Sports, 23/2 (2013), 171-80

20. Vesterinen, V. et al., 'Predictors of Individual Adaptation to High-volume or High-intensity Endurance training in Recreational Endurance Runners', Scandinavian Journal of Medicine and Science in Sports, 26/8 (2016), 885-93

Chapter 9: The Exercises

1. Schache, A., 'Eccentric Hamstring Muscle Training can Prevent Hamstring Injuries in Soccer Players', Journal of Physiotherapy, 58/1/58, (2012)

2. Timmins, R.G. et al., 'Biceps Femoris Architecture and Strength in Athletes with a Previous Anterior Cruciate Ligament Reconstruction'. Medicine & Science in Sports & Exercise, 48/3 (2016), 337

3. Brahler, C.J. and Blank, S.E., 'VersaClimbing Elicits Higher VO²max Than Does Treadmill Running or Rowing Ergometry', Medicine and Science in Sports and Exercise, 27/2 (1995), 249-54

Chapter 11: The 8-week Training Programme

1. Gabel, K. et al., 'Effects of 8-Hour Time Restricted Feeding on Body Weight and Metabolic Disease Risk Factors in Obese Adults: A Pilot Study', Nutrition and Healthy Aging, 4/4 (2018), 345

2. Atherton et al., 'Muscle Protein Synthesis in Response to Nutrition and Exercise', Journal of Physiology; 590/5 (2012), 1049

3. McLeay, Y. et al., 'Effect of New Zealand Blueberry Consumption on Recovery from Eccentric Exercise-induced Muscle Damage', Journal of the International Society of Sports Nutrition, 9/1 (2012), 19

4. Krikorian, R. et al., 'Blueberry Supplementation Improves Memory in Older Adults', Journal of Agriculture and Food Chemistry, 58/7 (2010)

5. Wu, T. et al., 'Blueberry and Mulberry Juice Prevent Obesity Development in C57BL/6 Mice', PLoS One, 8/10 (2013), e77585

6. Federation of American Societies for Experimental Biology, 'Blueberries May Inhibit Development of Fat Cells', Science Daily, (2011)

7. Qin, C. et al. on behalf of the China Kadoorie Biobank Collaborative Group, 'Associations of Egg Consumption with Cardiovascular Disease in a Cohort Study of 0.5 Million Chinese Adults', Heart, (2018)

8. Ho, K.Y. et al., 'Fasting Enhances Growth Hormone Secretion and Amplifies the Complex Rhythms of Growth Hormone Secretion in Man', Journal of Clinical Investigation, 81/4 (1988), 968-75

9. Röjdmark, S. et al., 'Pituitary-Testicular Axis in Obese Men During Short-Term Fasting', Acta Endocrinologica, 121/5 (1989), 727-32

10. Schanke, W. et al., 'Top 3 Most Effective Chest Exercises', ACE Certified News, (2012)

11. Berryman, C.E., et al., 'Inclusion of Almonds in a Cholesterol-Lowering Diet Improves Plasma HDL Subspecies and Cholesterol Efflux to Serum in Normal-Weight Individuals with Elevated LDL Cholesterol', Journal of Nutrition, 147/8 (2017), 1517-1523

12. Tang, G. et al., 'Meta-Analysis of the Association Between Whole Grain Intake and Coronary Heart Disease Risk', American Journal of Cardiology, 115/5 (2015), 625-9

Author's acknowledgements

Thank you to everyone at Bloomsbury who has worked on this book, most particularly for the input of Matthew Lowing and Zoë Blanc, you've been a joy to work with guys. I'd like to thank Peta, whom I've known for what feels like forever. It's great to (finally) work on a book together, having done so many pieces for newspapers over the last (20!) years! Mostly, I'd like to thank Jon, my brother, without whom this book simply wouldn't exist. His research and writing are the nuts and bolts of what you are reading and he's very much the unsung, untitled hero of the hour, so thank you!

Publisher's acknowledgements

The publisher would like to thank Josh Gardner and the whole team at Matt Roberts Personal Training; Yvonne Roberts; and Kings Cross Estates for permission to use their locations for photography.

Graphic Design: Blok Graphic, London.
Models: Tino Clarke and Martin Miller at Base Model Management.
Clothing: Matt Roberts' workout clothing was provided by Descente.

Index

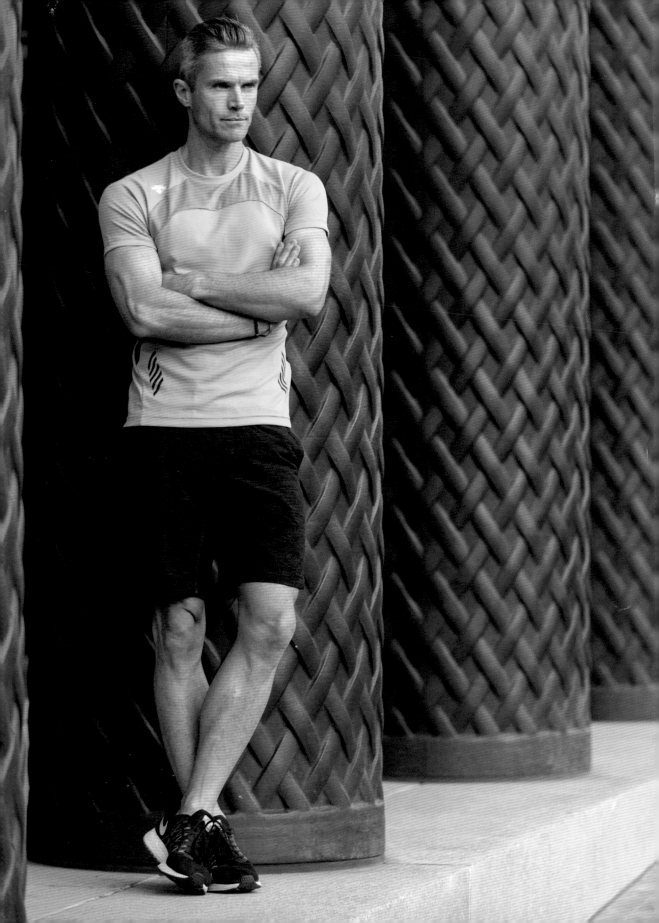